Book VALUES

connection
responsibility
economical
practical
access
life
fairness
sustainability
empowerment
nutrition
education
interaction
maximising potential
health
modelling
wholefood
longevity
seasonality
consistency
appreciation
equity
realistic
credibility

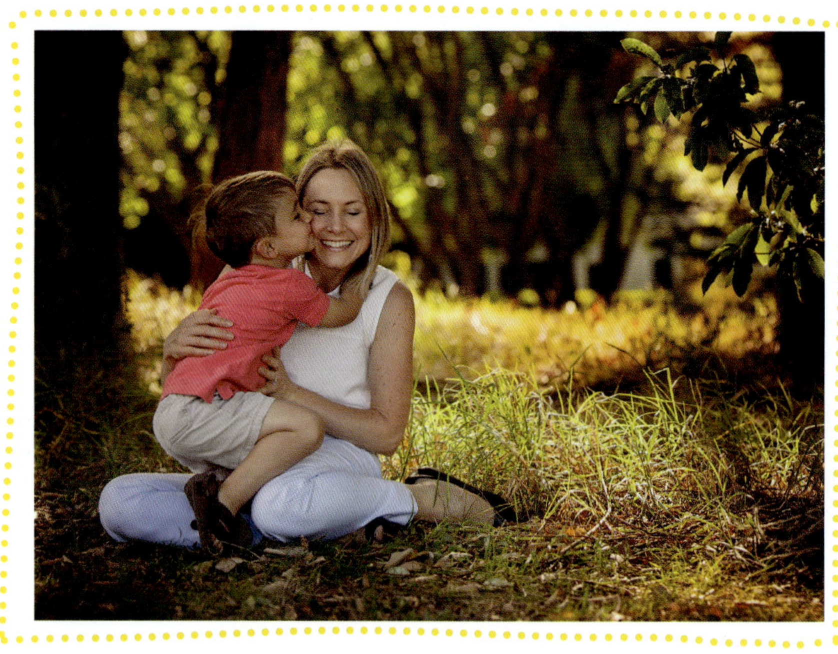

About BITE NUTRITION and the author

Bite Nutrition was created to offer practical, simple, beautiful books and tools to help carers, parents and educators get their children interested in their health and nutrition.

After years of working with adults as a Dietitian, the founder and author, Tanya Nagy decided she wanted to focus on educating humans when they were much younger; with no doubt that so much of who we are as adults is from our very early years of life. Hence, the series "Feeding Growing Humans Beautiful Yummy Food" was created. To help towards introducing the best foods for growth and long term health and giving our children the best start we can.

A mother of 3 beautiful little ones, Tanya is keen to contribute and have a positive impact on the world. She believes we should all be more personally responsible for our behaviors and impact on the environment; with special consideration to sustainability, respect, kindness and paying it forward.

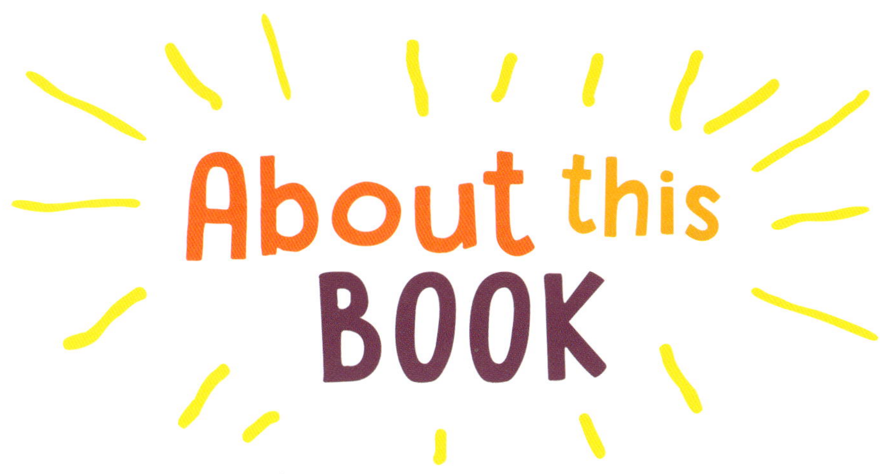

About this BOOK

You have this book because someone really **CARES** for you.
So, who gave you this book?

They want you to learn how to make **better choices** in the food you eat.

They want you to live a **LONG and HEALTHY Life** and be the **best that you can be.**

You are growing and as part of growing, your body needs helpful foods; foods that help you grow in a **healthy** way.

Sometimes what your body "needs" to be healthy and what you "want" because it tastes good can be different. Let's think of some examples of that.

Can YOU think of any?

This book is to show you real to life pictures of important foods that you need to learn about. It also tells you:

1. What **"season"** the food is best.
2. How the food **grows**.
3. How each **food is HELPFUL** to your body.
4. **How much** of each food you should eat each time and over the day.
5. A **recipe** for each food and some tips on how to shop for it and store it

Have fun learning about these **Beautiful Yummy Foods!** Then each day, let's try to choose what your body needs, most of the time!

What older readers SHOULD KNOW

This book is **NOT** designed to be an encyclopaedia of fruit. It has only some of the fruits we have to choose from. The fruits chosen, were chosen because they are one or a few of these following points:

1. Rich in **nutrition** (nutrient dense).
2. **Accessible** (i.e. volume, cost, found in most markets).
3. Can be used easily as **lunchbox/on the go** options.

want a fruit in the next book version?
contact us @

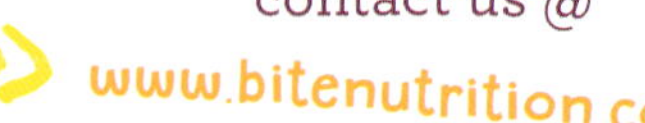

When you read to your younger learner, keep these things in mind.

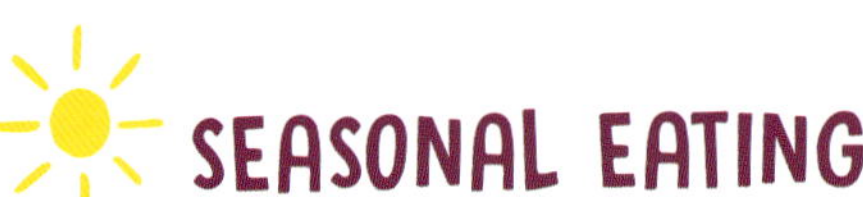

SEASONAL EATING

Choosing food in season is better for your health, the environment and your budget! Vitamins and minerals are at their highest in content in season. Also, the vitamins and minerals the foods in season have are those that your body needs the most at that time of year.

SEASONS KEY:

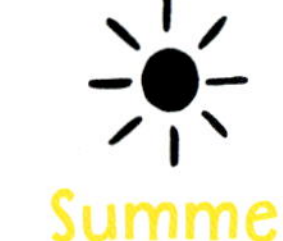

Summer
December, January, February

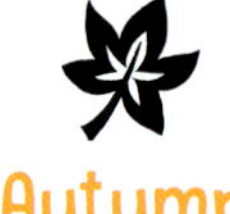

Autumn
March, April, May

Winter
June, July, August

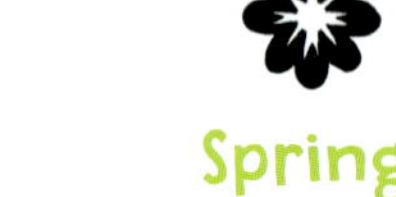

Spring
September, October, November

HOW FOOD IS GROWN

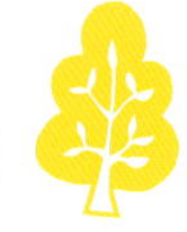

"Where does food come from?" *The shop?* It is important our children understand the food cycle and value the work our farmers do. Food takes a lot of effort to produce and learning about this will help them appreciate food more and hopefully, slowly, discourage them from wasting food!

SERVES AND VARIETY

Variety of food is so important for health. Too much of any food, even "healthy" food, is not helpful. Look at the colours in a rainbow and try to eat lots of colours, in foods, each day. There are many colours of fruits, so try to eat 2 colours each day in the right (total) serve size.

SERVES

Adults are recommended to have 2 serves of fruit **per day**. Children's needs are less:

1-2 yrs = ½ serve of fruit

2-3 yrs = 1 serve of fruit

4-8 yrs = 1 ½ serves of fruit

9-11+ yrs = 2 serves of fruit.

FRESH/FROZEN/CANNED/DRIED/BLENDED

What is best!? **Fresh in season is best** where you can. Next best is snap frozen, canned, blended then dried. Whole fresh fruit, skin on where possible, is always going to be better for you.

VITAMINS AND MINERALS—TRYING TO KEEP THEM

- Always wash your fruit before eating it.
- Do not peel your fruit if you can avoid it; unless the skin is not edible, like banana skin, orange peel or mango skin. The skin has lots of great fibre to help your tummy and there are lots of vitamins just under the skin you may peel away. You can eat kiwi fruit skin! Try it!!
- Try not to chop up your fruit too much. The vitamins inside break very easily and lots of chopping is not helpful in keeping the vitamins.
- As soon as you start to heat fruit, the vitamins and minerals inside will start to disappear. Fruit is best fresh. If you do cook fruit, try to atleast keep the skin on so you get the fibre.

THE IMPORTANCE OF WATER

An average of 70% of your body is water. Plain, clean water helps your body; including getting oxygen to your brain so you can think, concentrate, learn and be at your full potential. Other fluids are not as helpful. More water please!!!

BEES

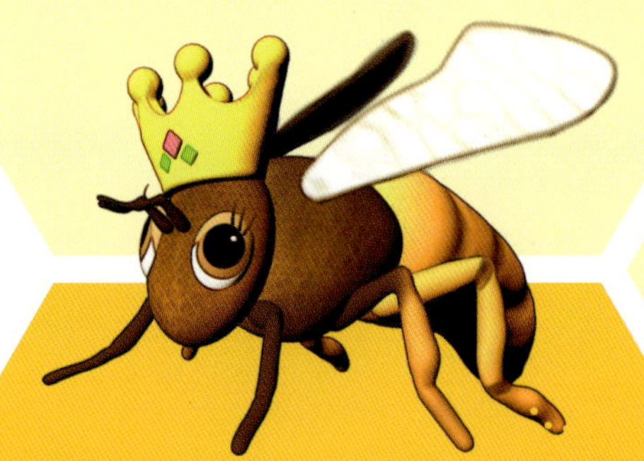

ORLA

is a QUEEN BEE

Each bee hive has a queen and a colony of worker and drone bee's. Worker bees are girls and drone bees are boys. Each colony would have at least 20,000 bees or more!

Bees are so very important in making the food that we eat; for making crops that are used for clothes we wear, like cotton, and our environment. The worker bees **"pollinate"** so that our foods can grow.

Every third mouthful of food is a food that could grow thanks to bee's.

Please learn more about bees and take care of them. They are very **precious**.

Bee's also help feed our native wildlife, help feed our cows and other animals that are in our food supply. Not to mention they make **yummy honey**!!

You will find Orla on pages where she is needed to make the fruit.

Look for her!

Quote for older readers:

"The way humanity manages or mismanages its nature-based assets, including pollinators, will in part define our collective future in the 21st century... The fact is that of the 100 crop species that provide 90 percent of the worlds food, over 70 are pollinated by bee's".

Achim Steiner.
Executive Director UN Environmental Program 2006-2016

How to READ this BOOK

TODDLERS

1. Look at the pictures
2. Learn to recognize the fruit
3. Look for Orla

PRESCHOOLERS

1. Learn which season its best
2. Learn where it grows
3. Learn how the food can help you
4. Learn what a serve size is
5. Talk about eating fresh fruit each day

SCHOOL KIDS

1. Pick one fruit each week
2. Look at the recipe and go shopping for it
3. Practice how to choose and store the fruit
4. Then prepare the recipe and eat!

YOU CAN ALSO...

1. Learn how important bees are to our environment
2. Learn the book values and add some of your own
3. Do the quiz at the back!

BERRIES

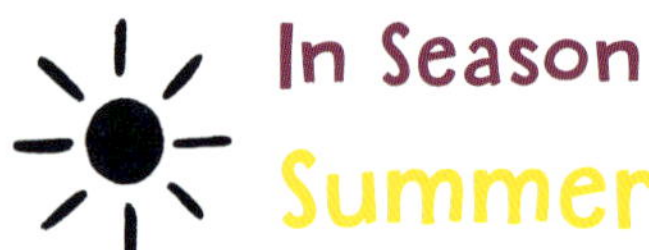

In Season

Summer

Grows How?

On bushes

A Serve

1/2 cup

Good For Your

heart

bones

strength

brain

tummy

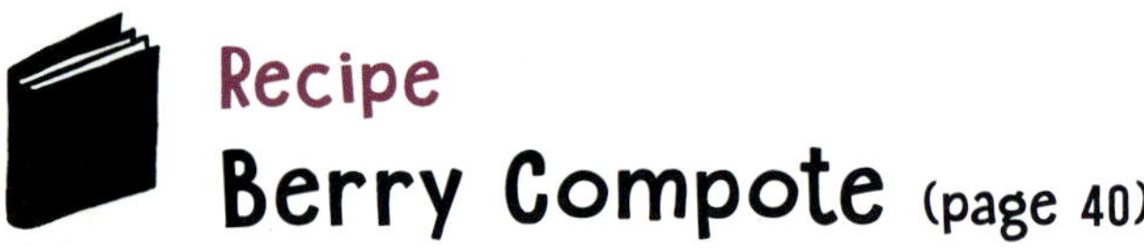

Recipe

Berry Compote (page 40)

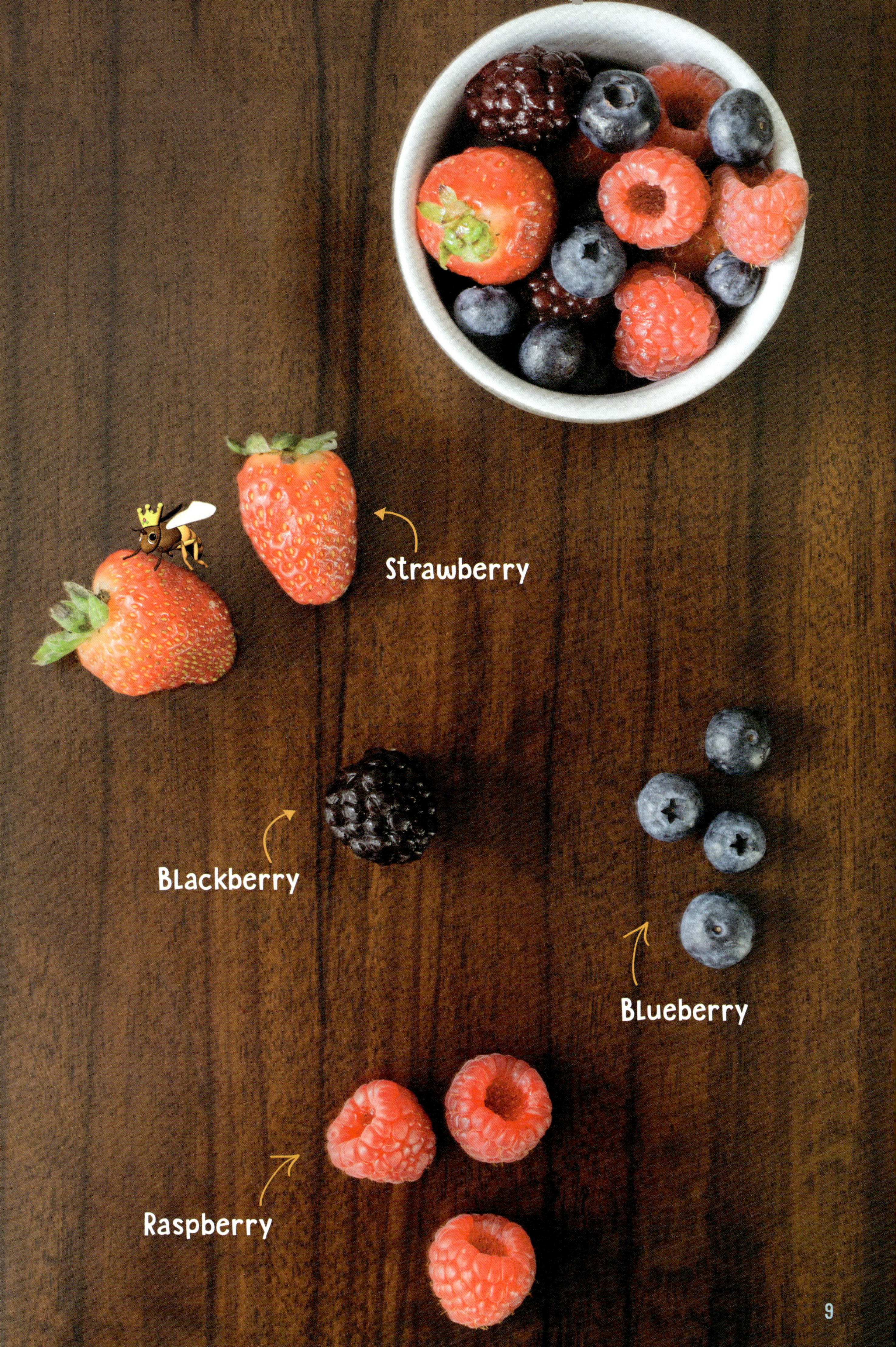
Strawberry
Blackberry
Blueberry
Raspberry

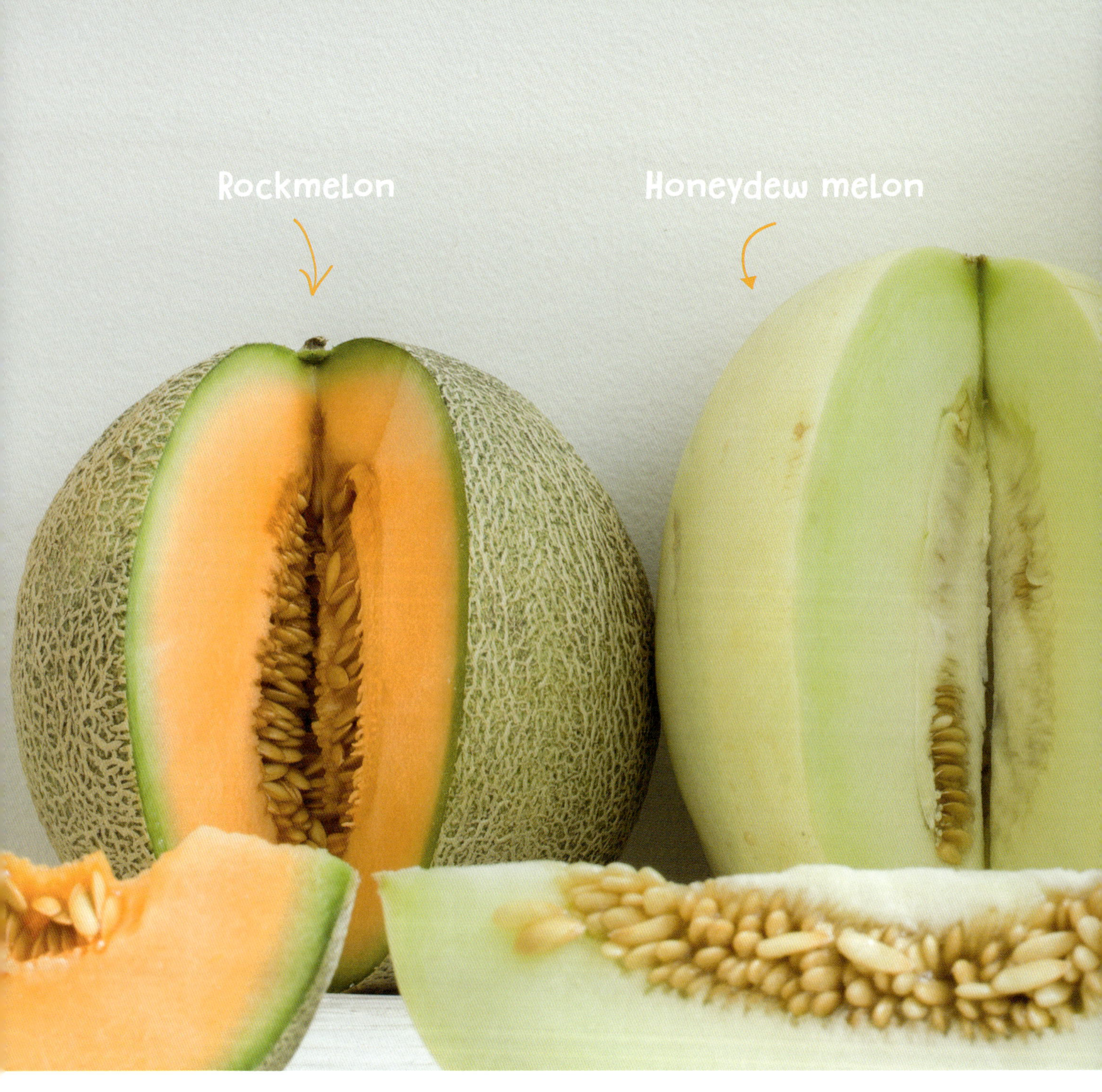

MELON

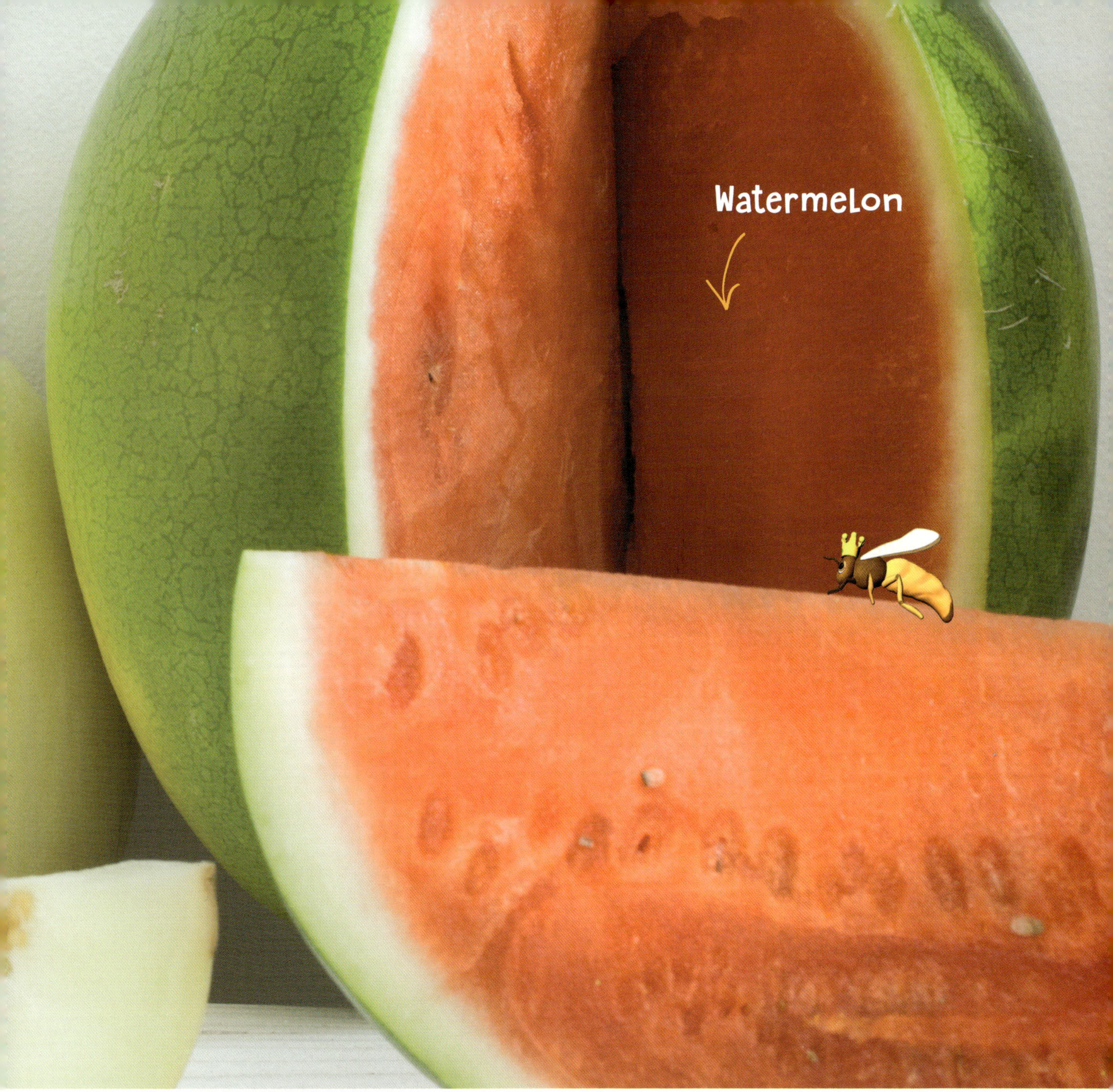

Watermelon

In Season
Summer

Grows How?
On vines

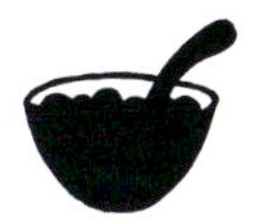

A Serve
1 cup

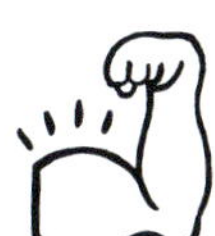

Good For Your
strength

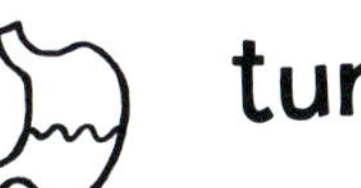

tummy

energy

eyes
(rockmelon)

Recipe
Watermelon Salad (page 43)

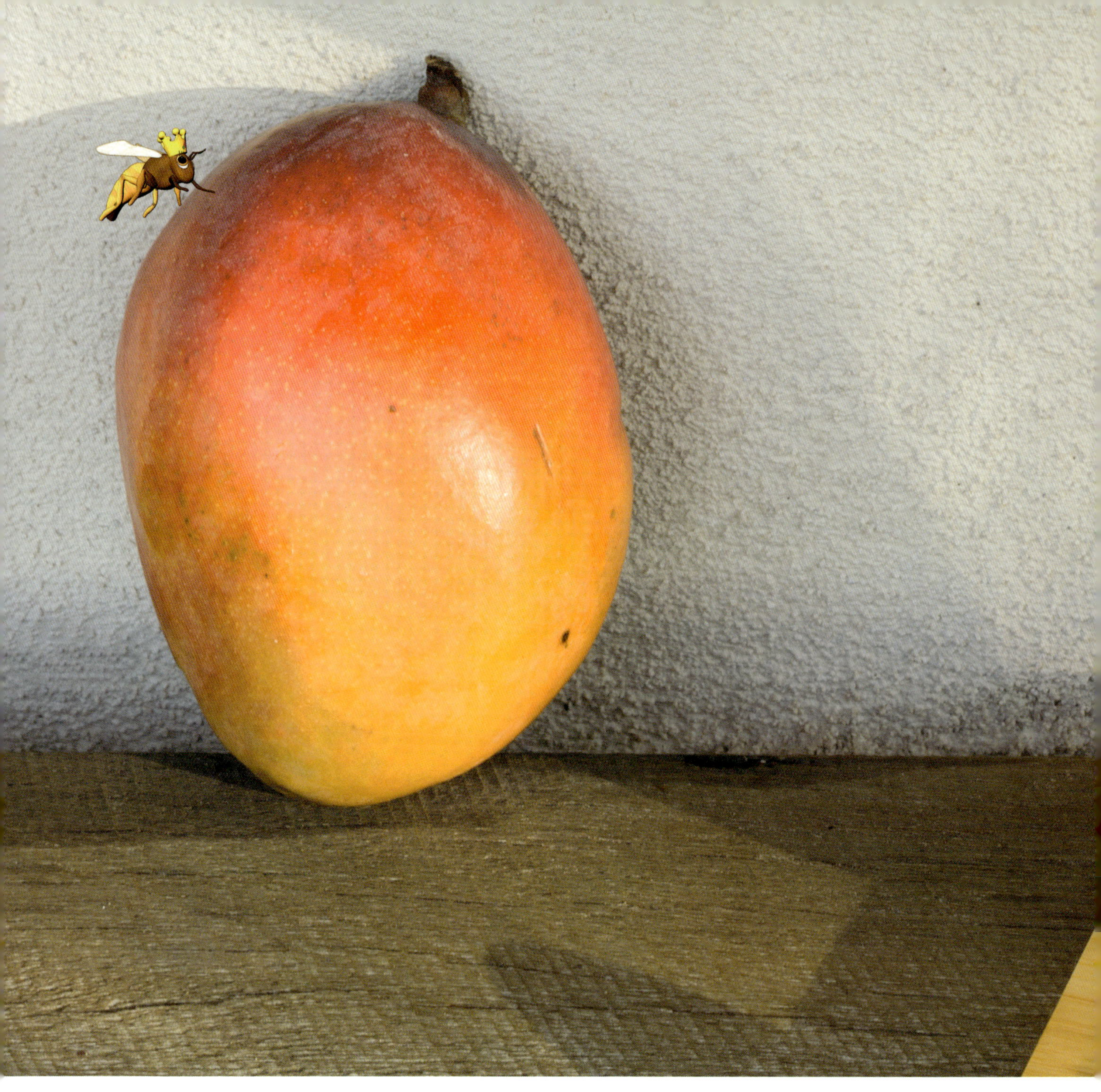

MANGO

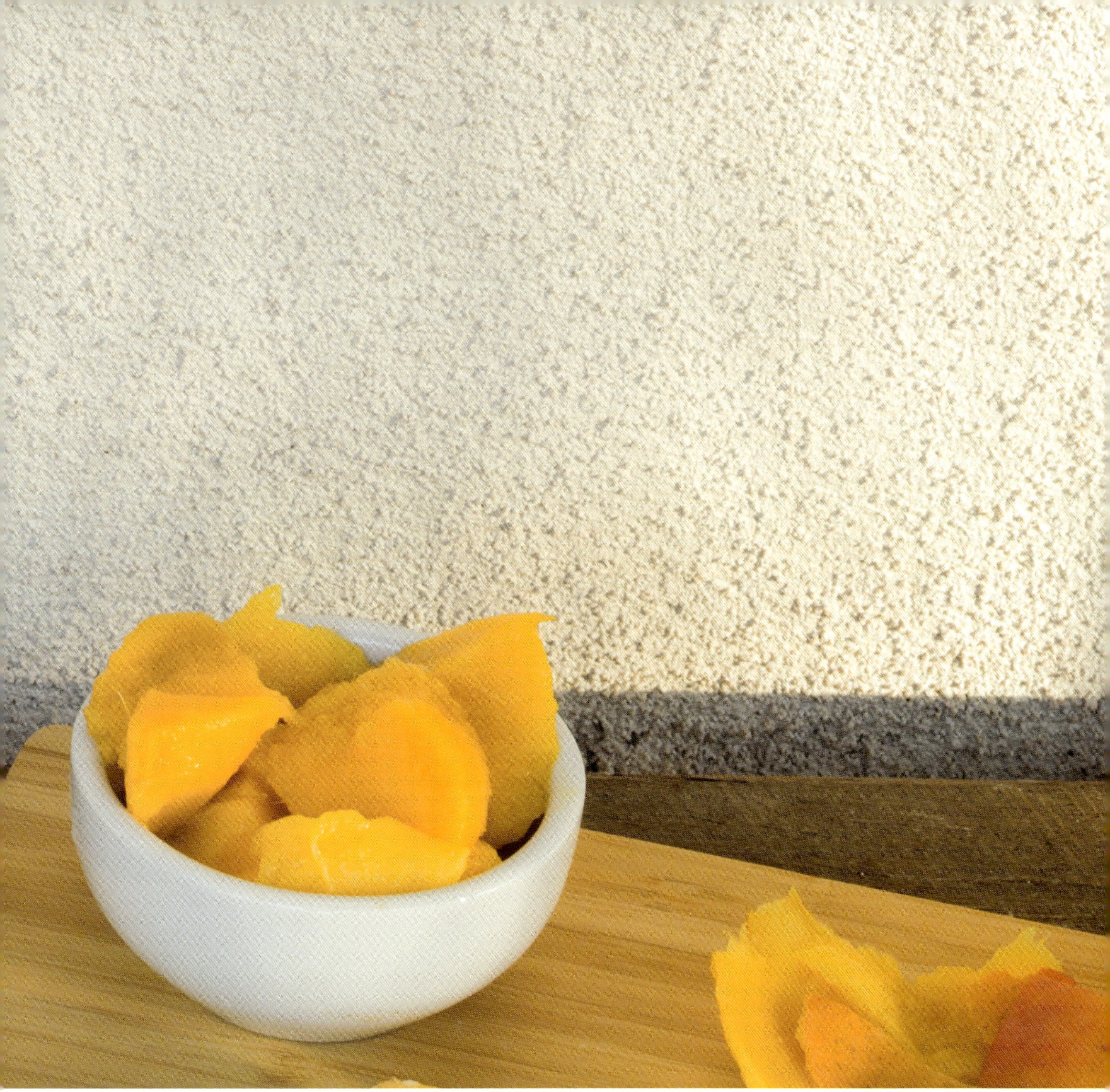

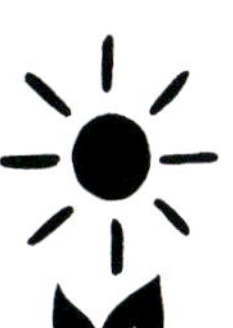

In Season
Summer

and Autumn

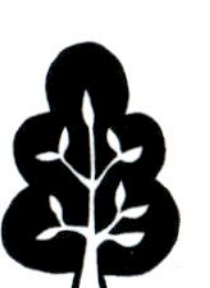

Grows How?
In trees

A Serve
1 medium mango

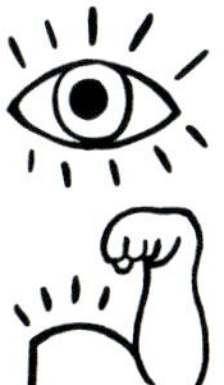

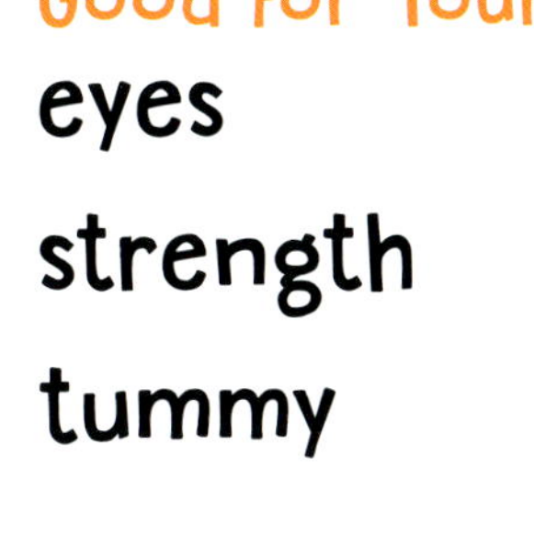

Good For Your
eyes
strength
tummy

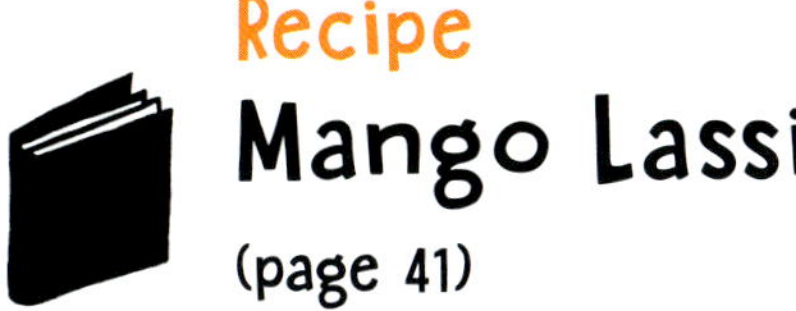

Recipe
Mango Lassi
(page 41)

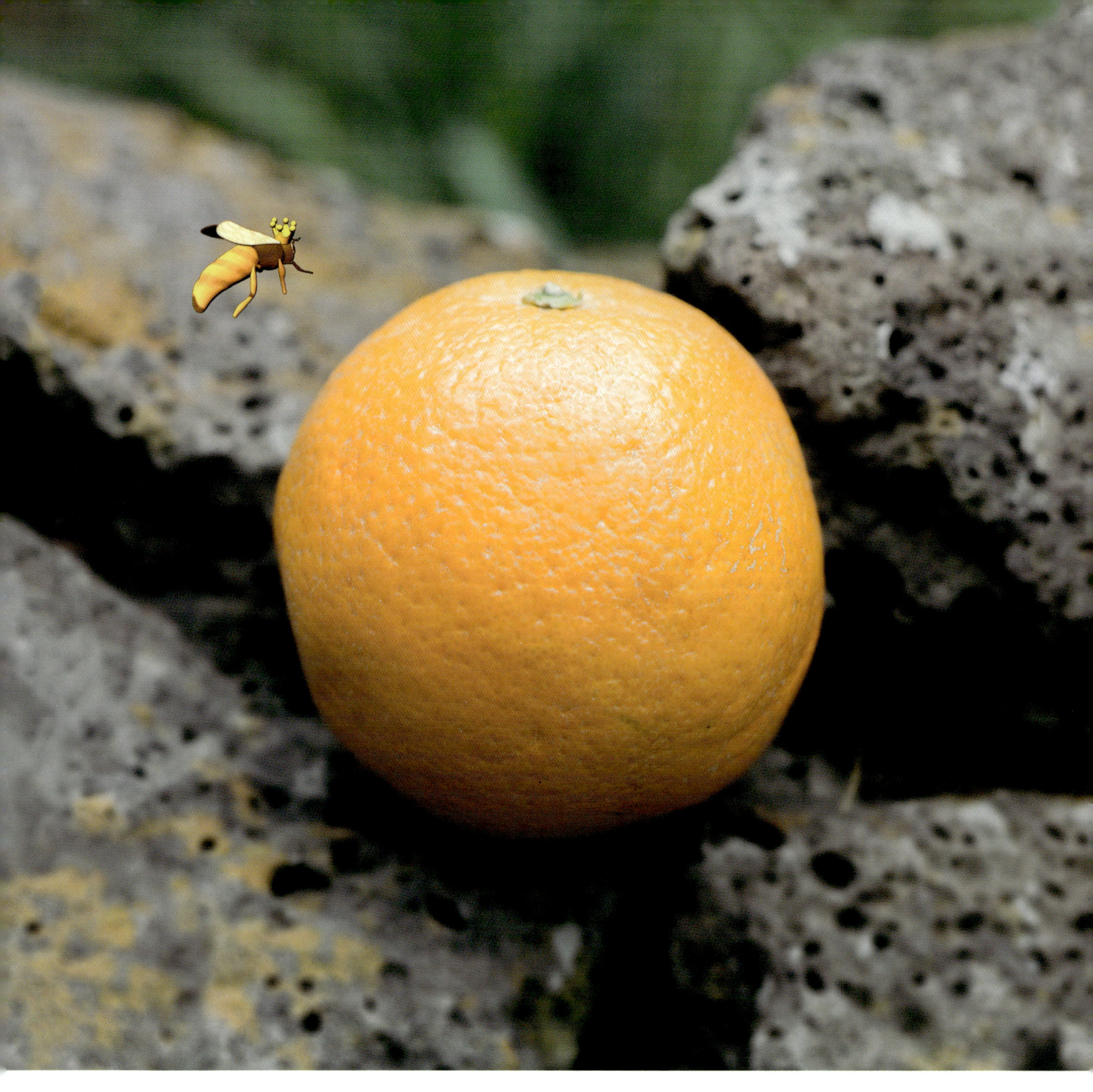

ORANGE

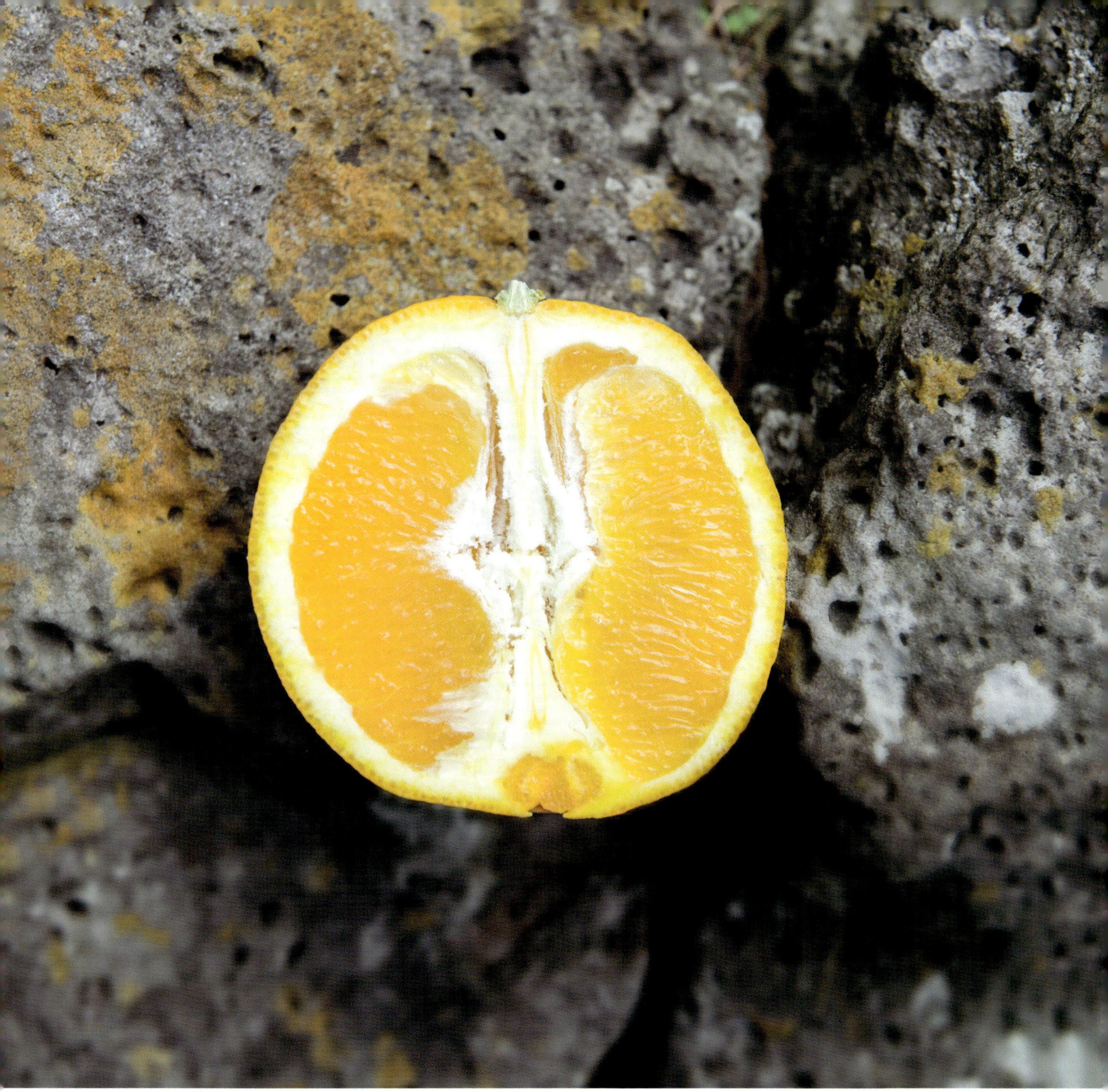

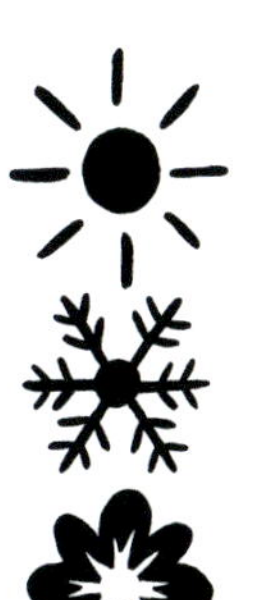

In Season

Summer (Valencia)

Winter and Spring (Navel)

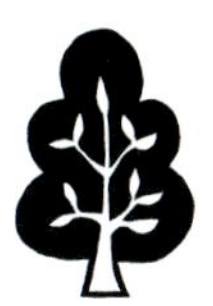

Grows How?

In trees

A Serve

1 orange

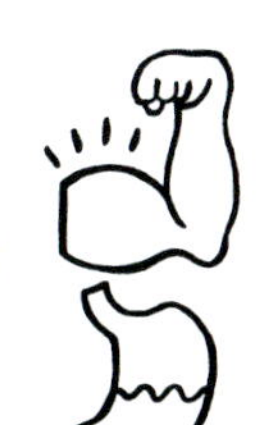

Good For Your

strength

tummy

energy

heart

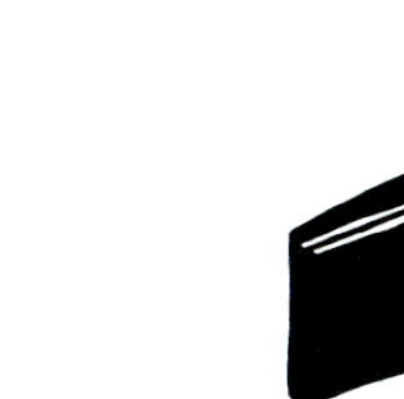

Recipe

Orange and Beetroot salad (page 41)

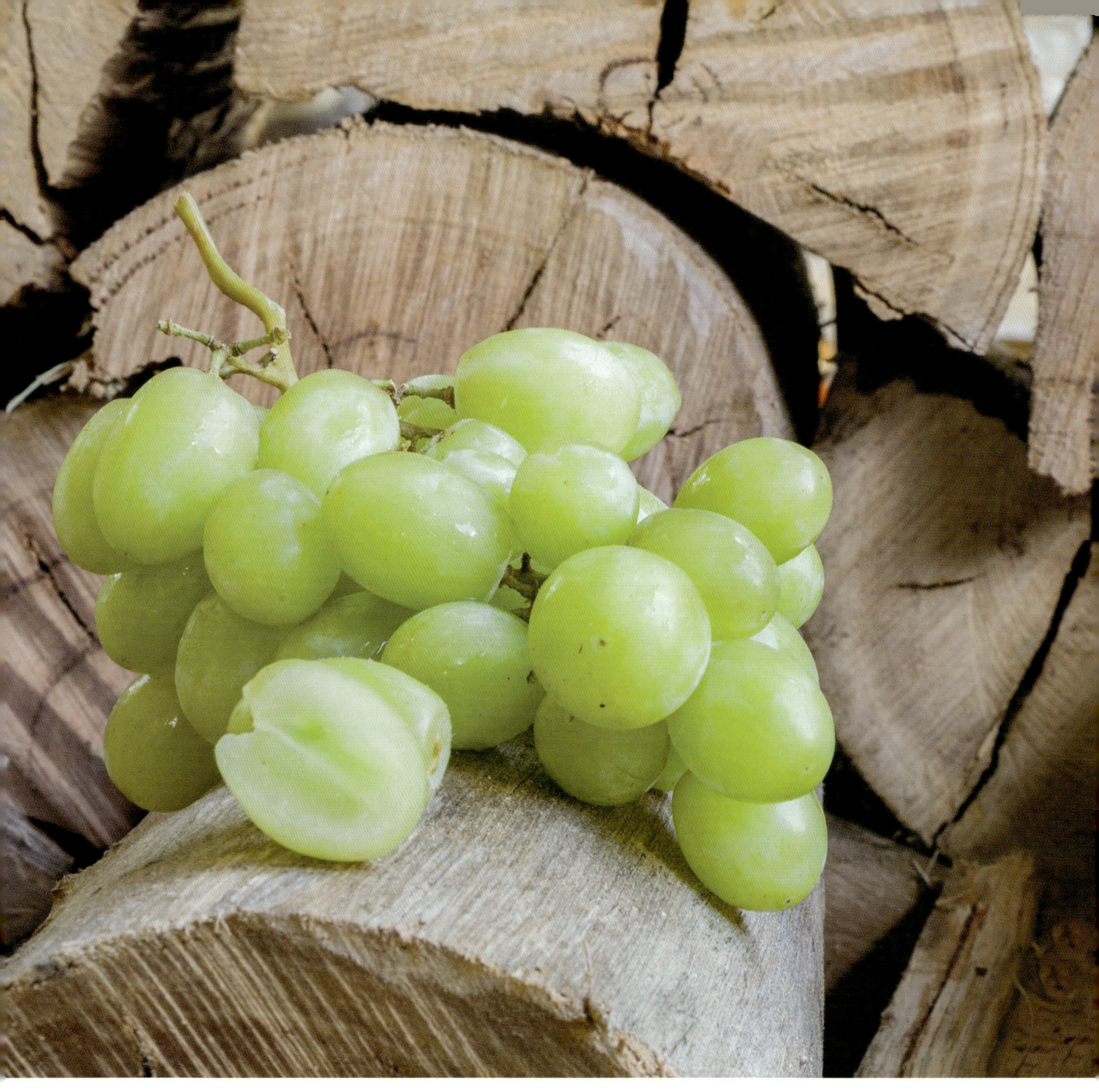

GRAPES

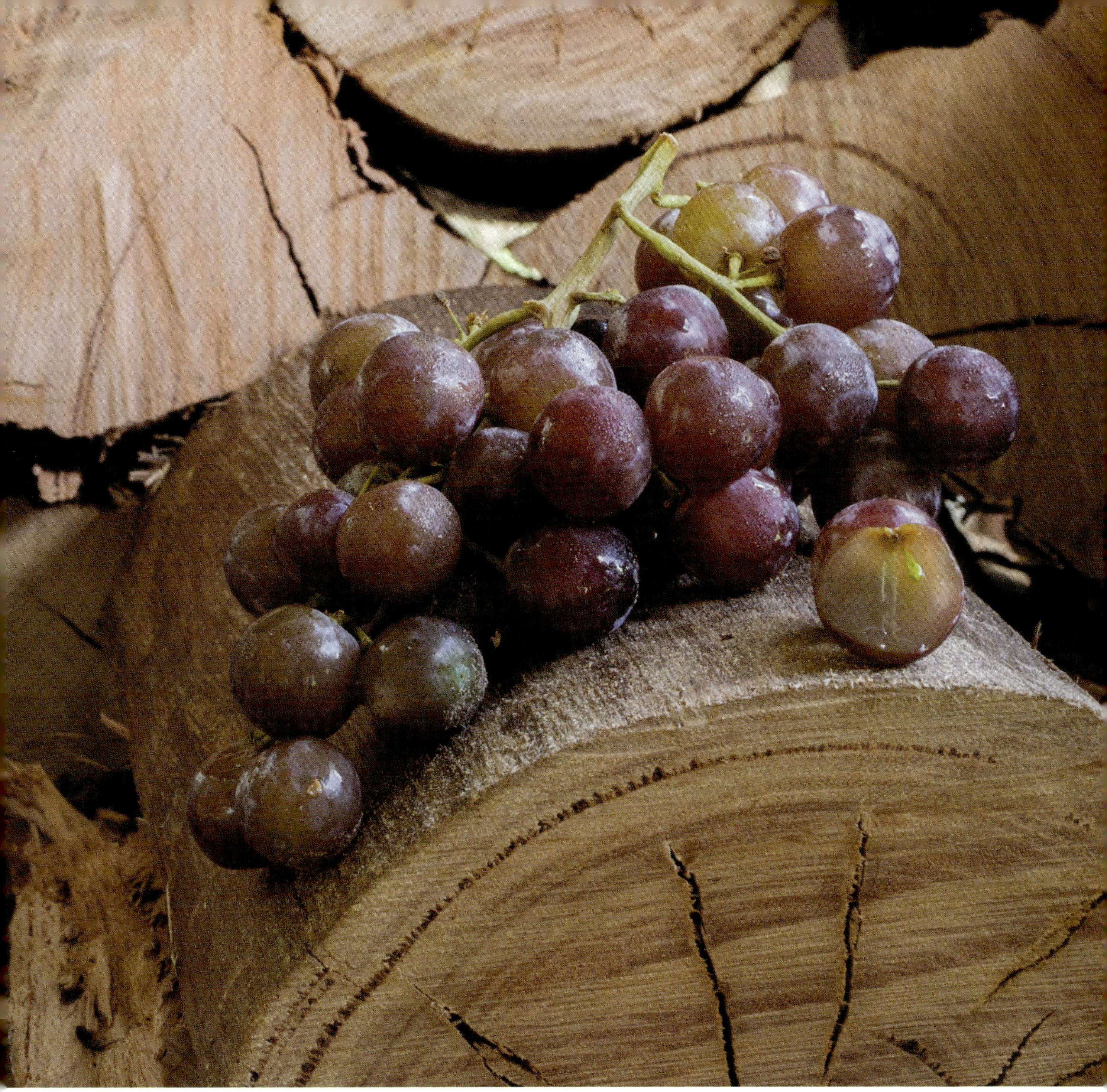

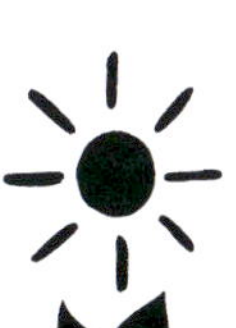

In Season
Summer

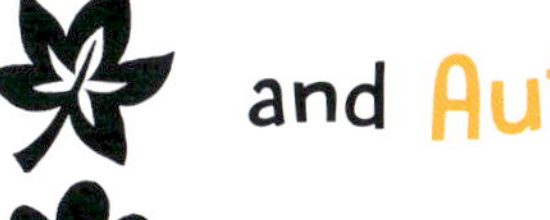

and Autumn

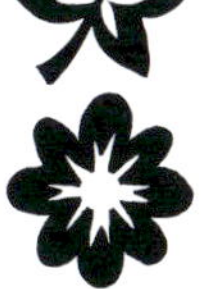

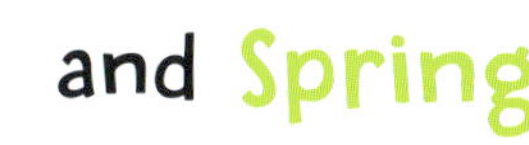

and Spring

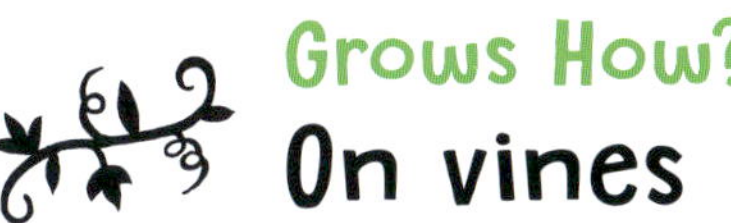

Grows How?
On vines

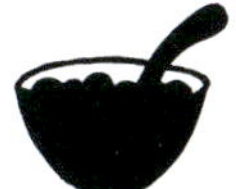

A Serve
10 grapes

Good For Your
heart

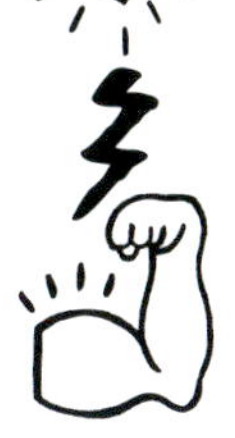

energy

strength

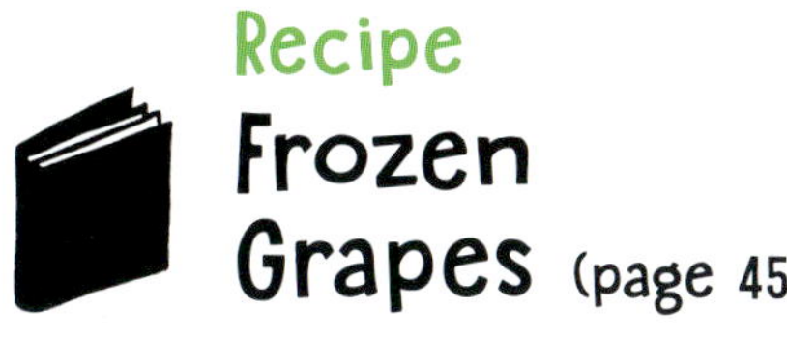

Recipe
Frozen Grapes (page 45)

CHERRY

In Season

Summer

and

Spring

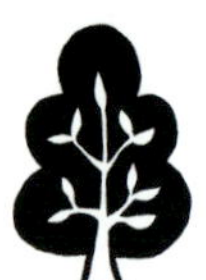

Grows How?

In trees

A Serve

10 cherries

Good For Your

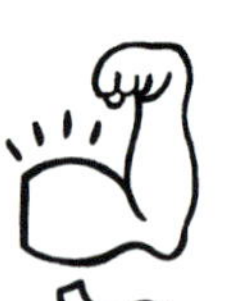

strength

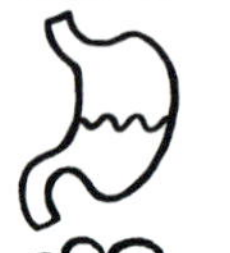

tummy

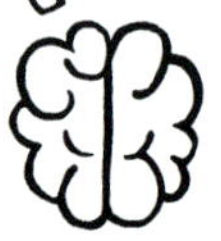

brain

heart

Recipe

Cherry Salad (page 42)

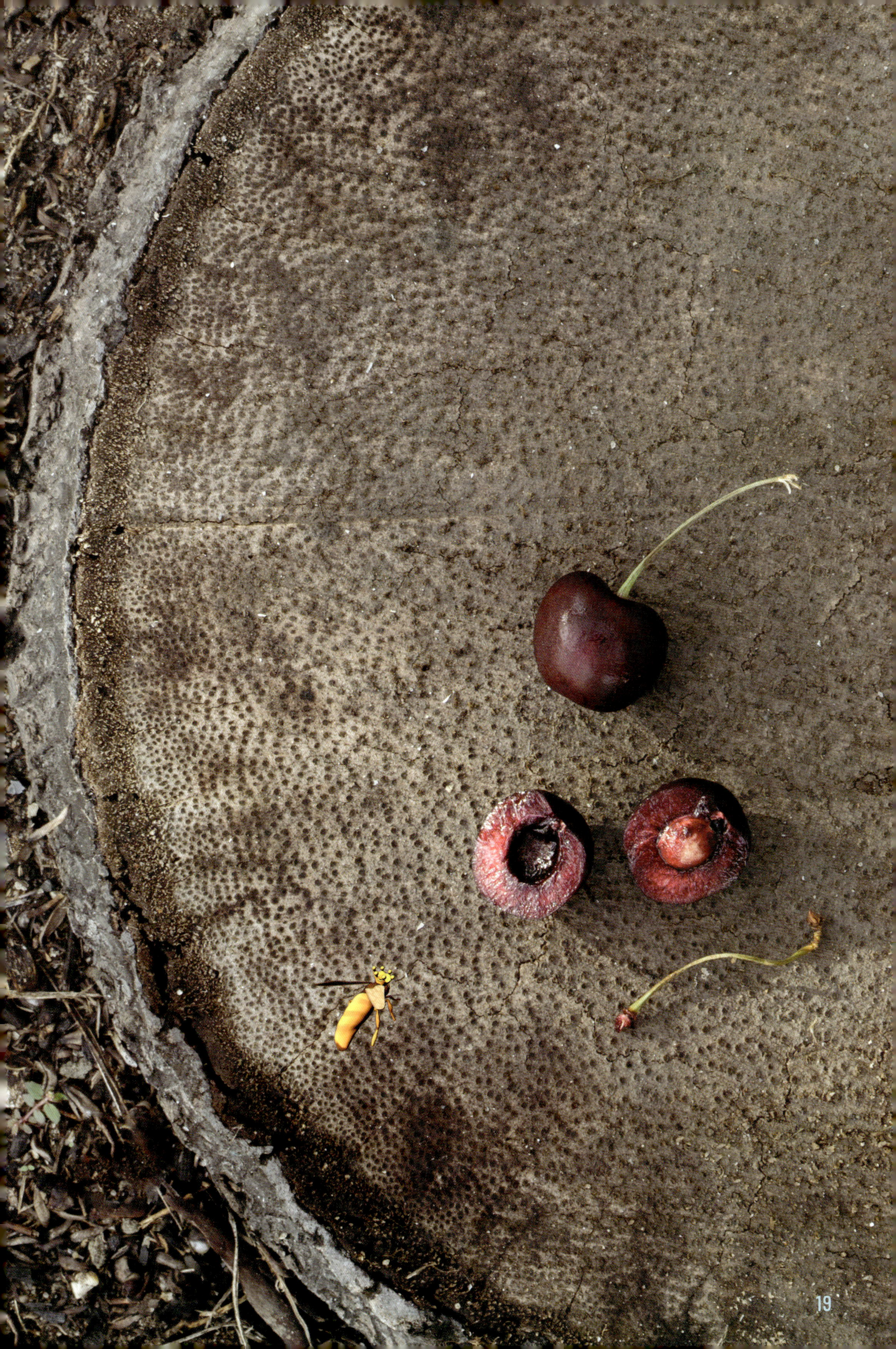

STONE FRUIT

In Season

Summer

and

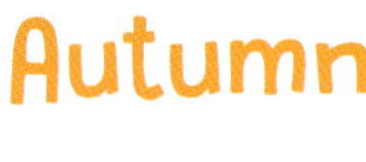

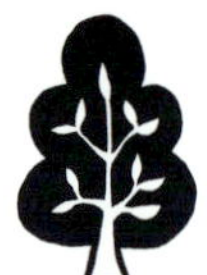

Grows How?

In trees

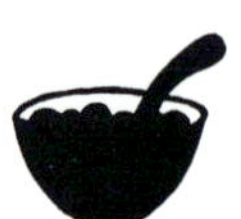

A Serve

2 small or 1 large

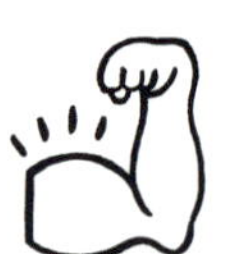

Good For Your

strength

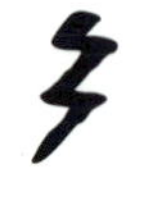

energy

heart

Recipe

Nectarine and Yoghurt Slice (page 39)

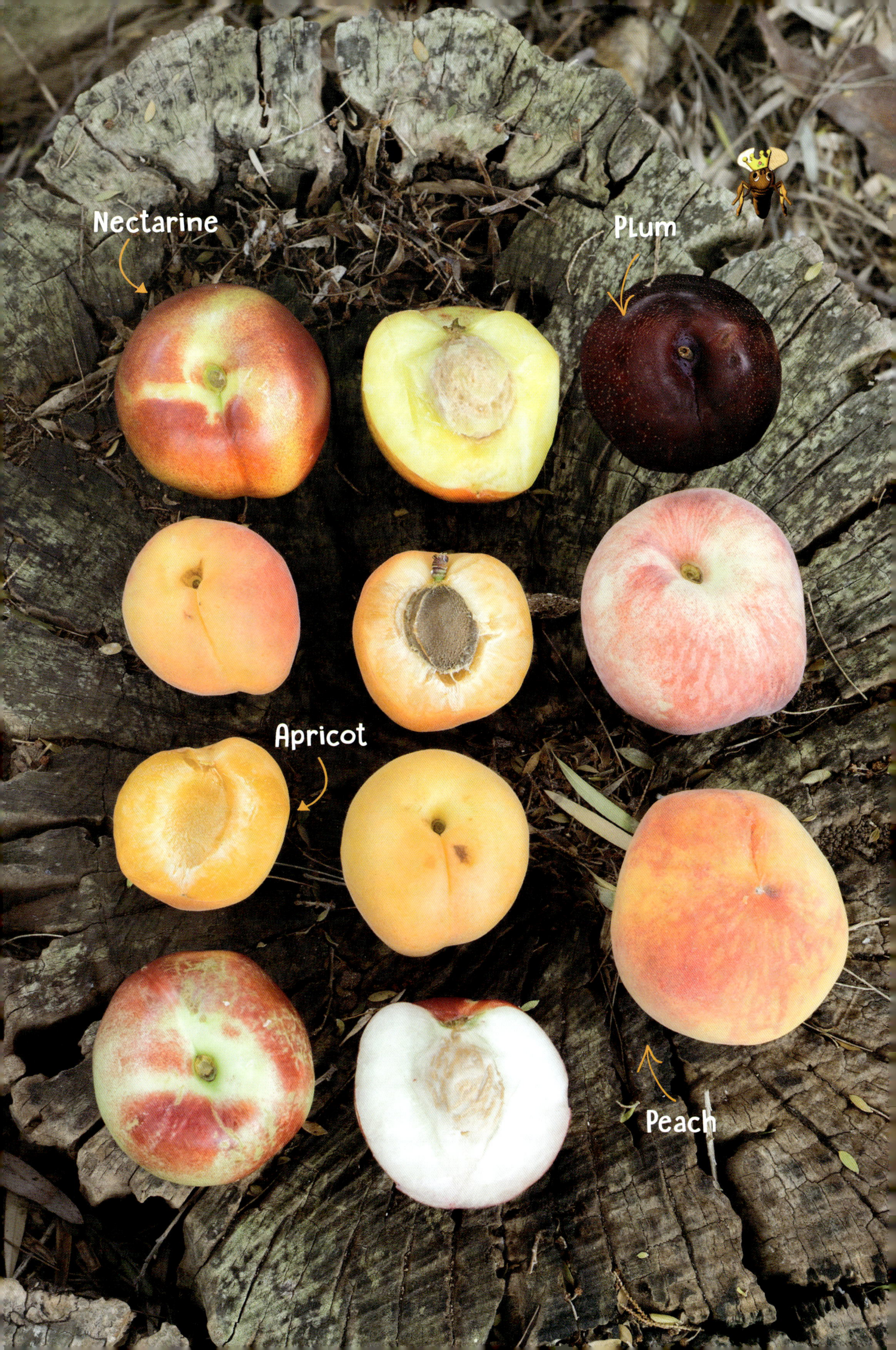
Nectarine
Plum
Apricot
Peach

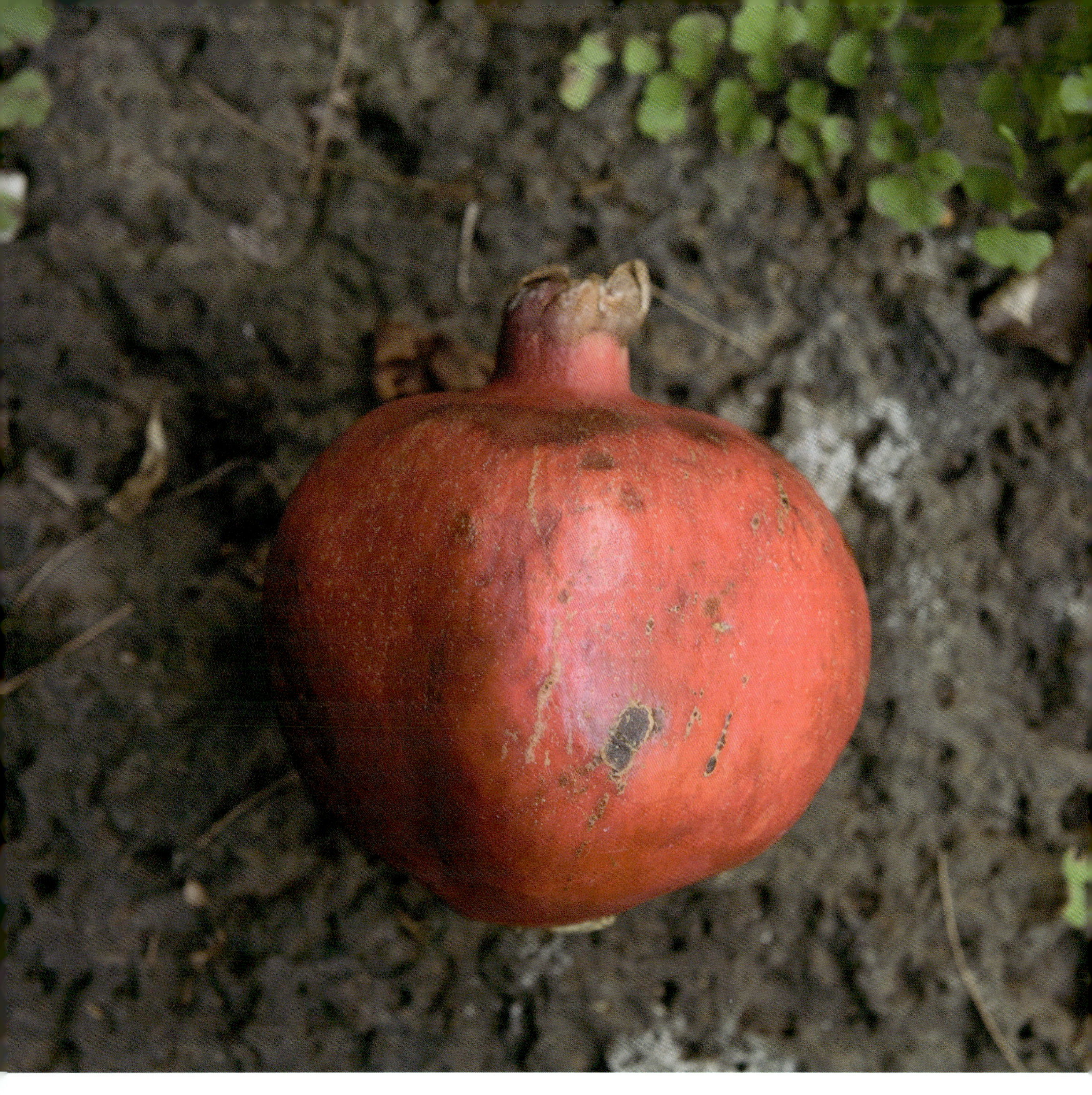

POMEGRANATE

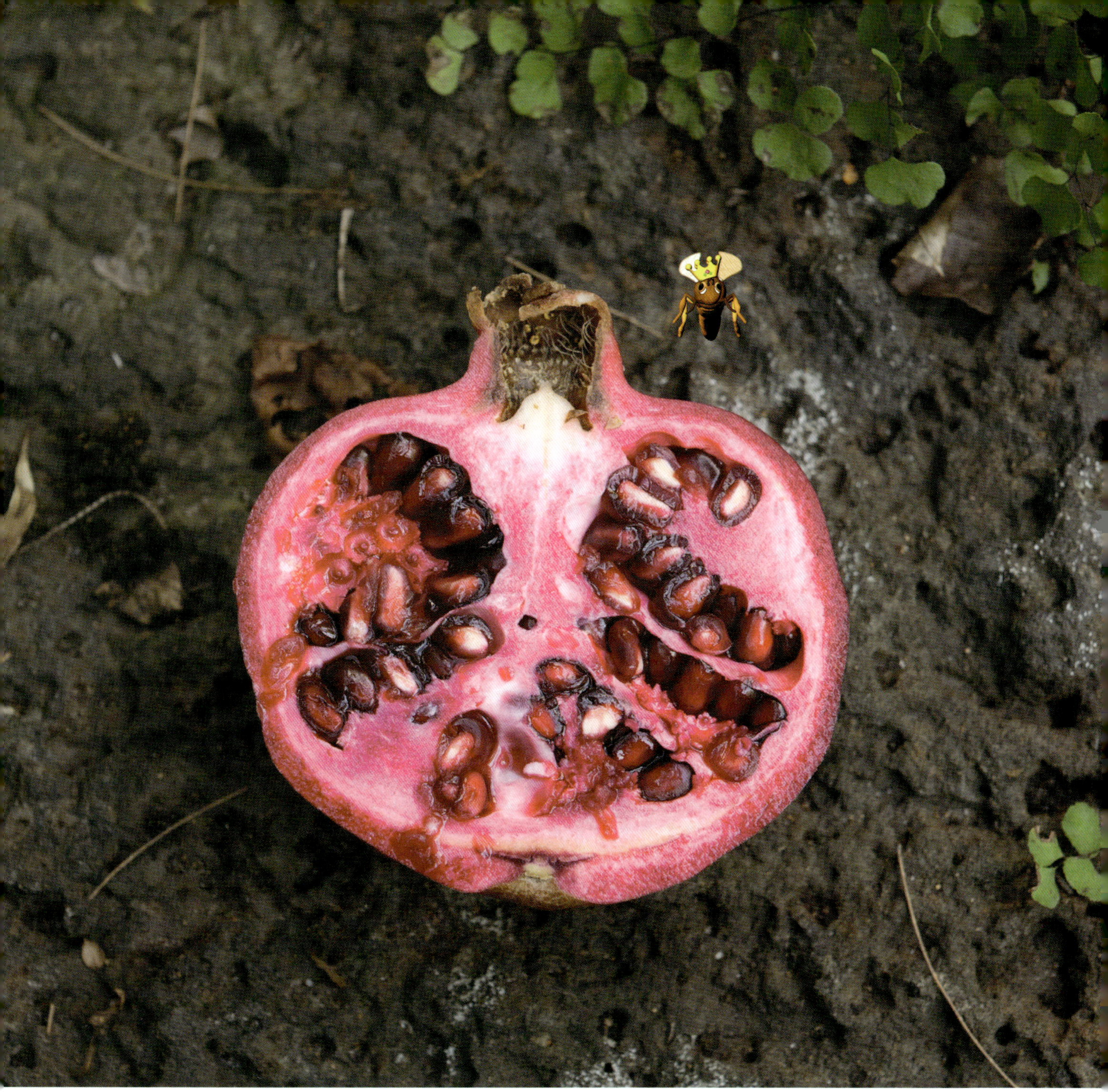

In Season
Autumn

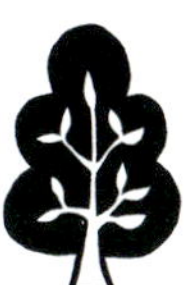

Grows How?
In trees

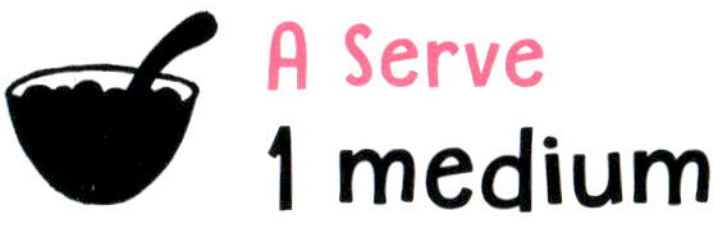

A Serve
1 medium

Good For Your

heart

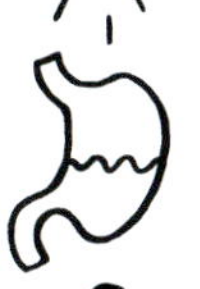

tummy

energy

Recipe

Bulger and Pomegranate Salad (page 44)

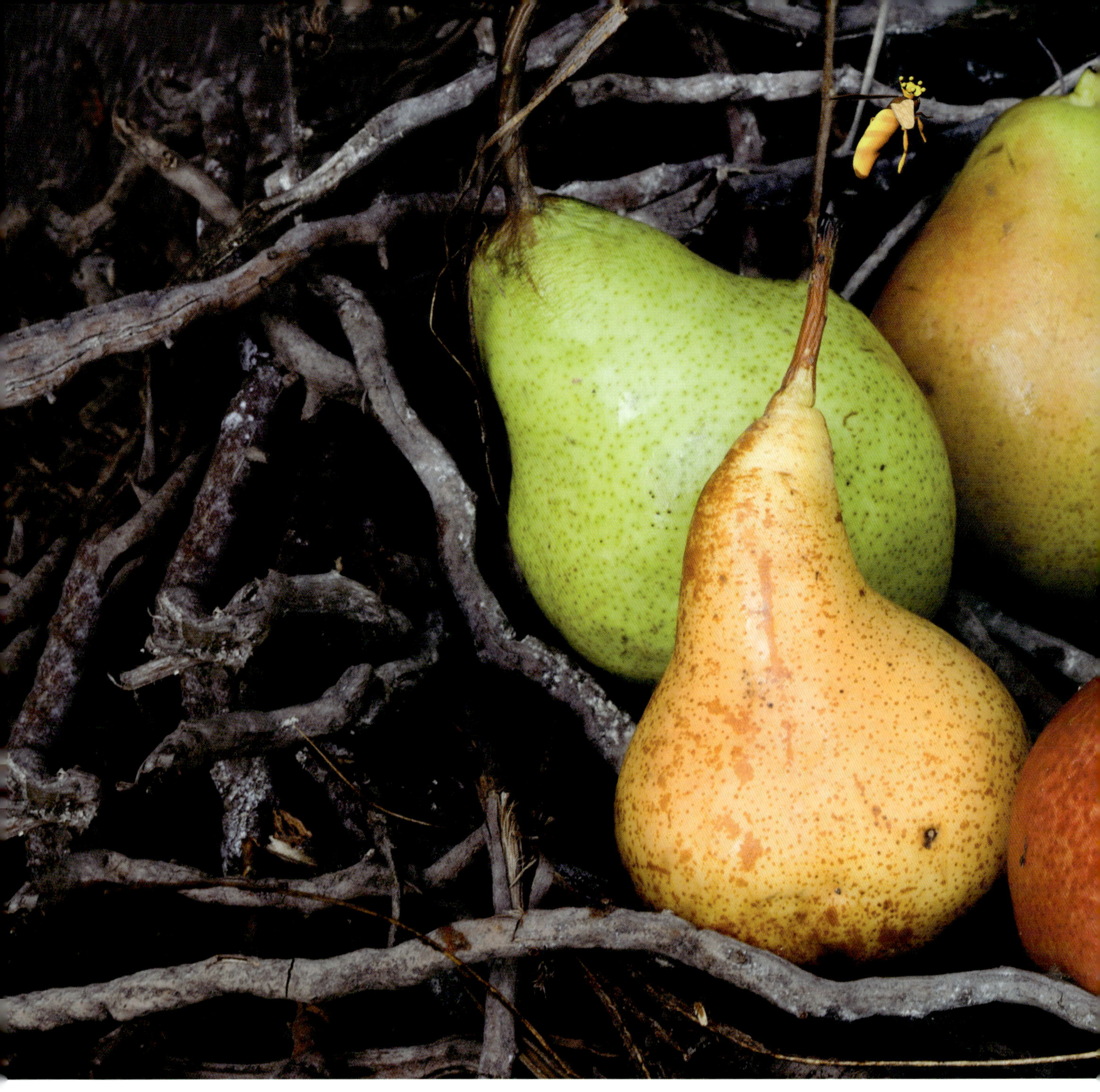

PEARS

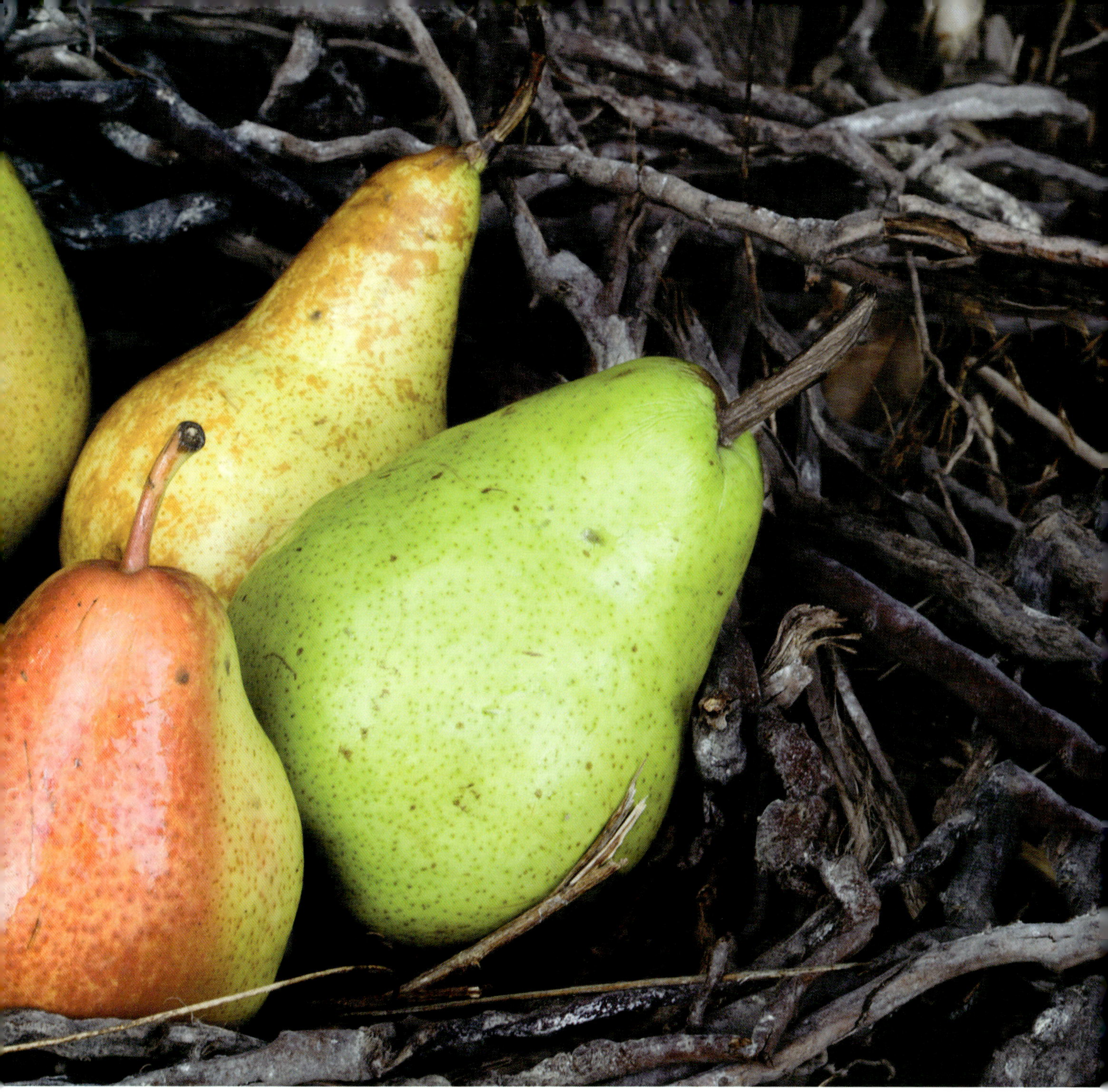

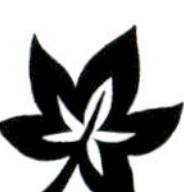

In Season
Autumn

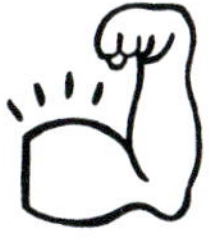

Good For Your
strength

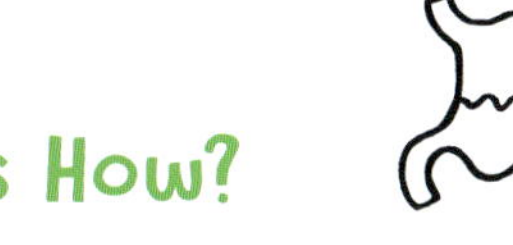

tummy

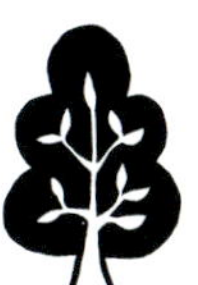

Grows How?
In trees

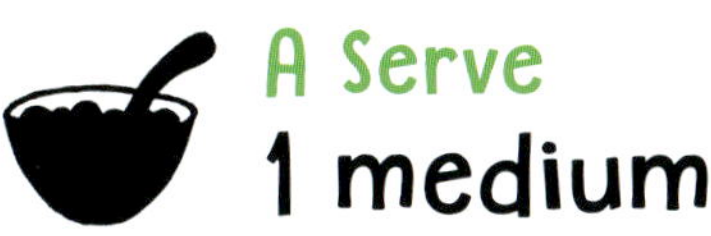

A Serve
1 medium

Recipe
Pear, Walnut and Pumpkin Salad (page 43)

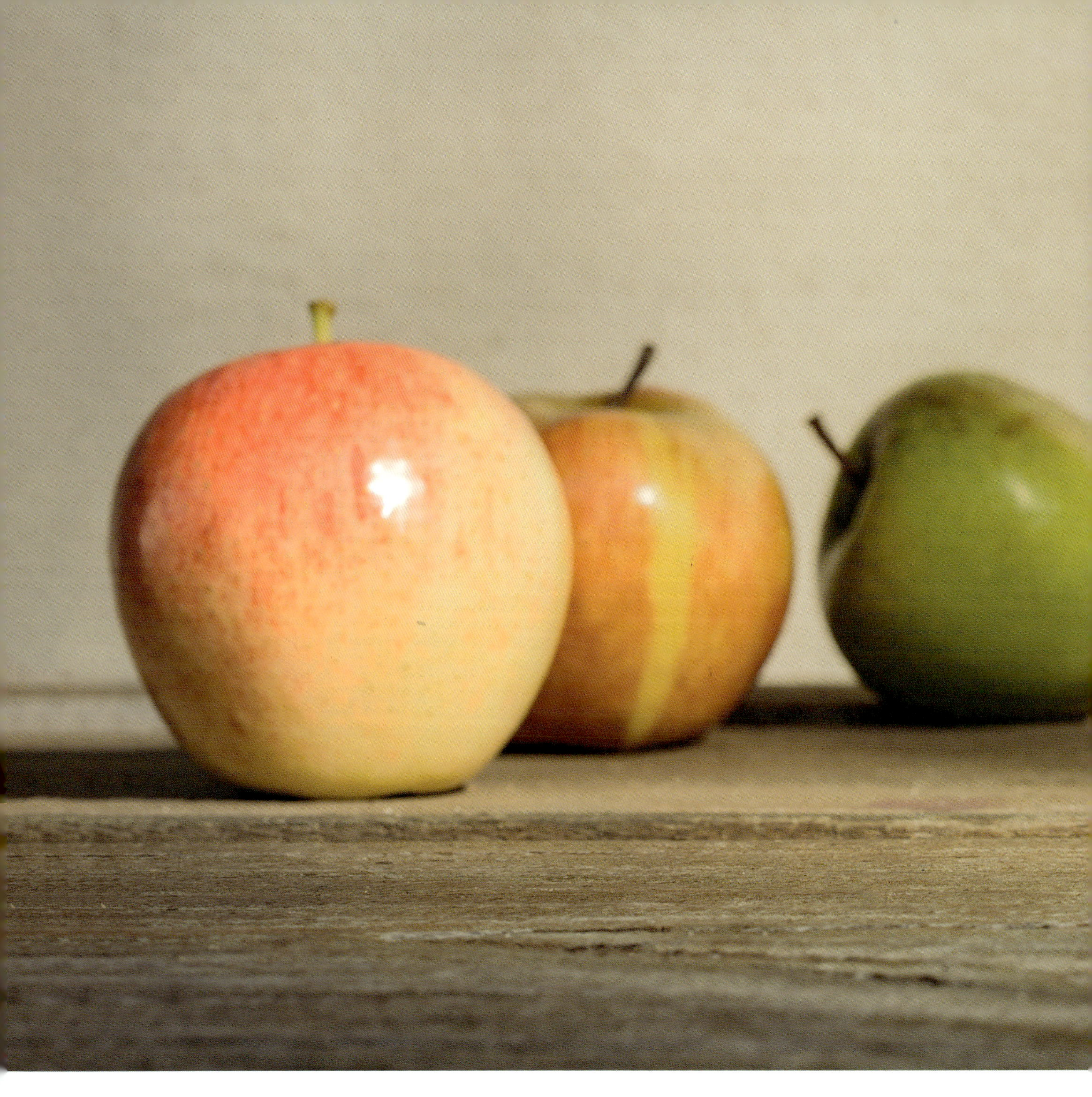

APPLES

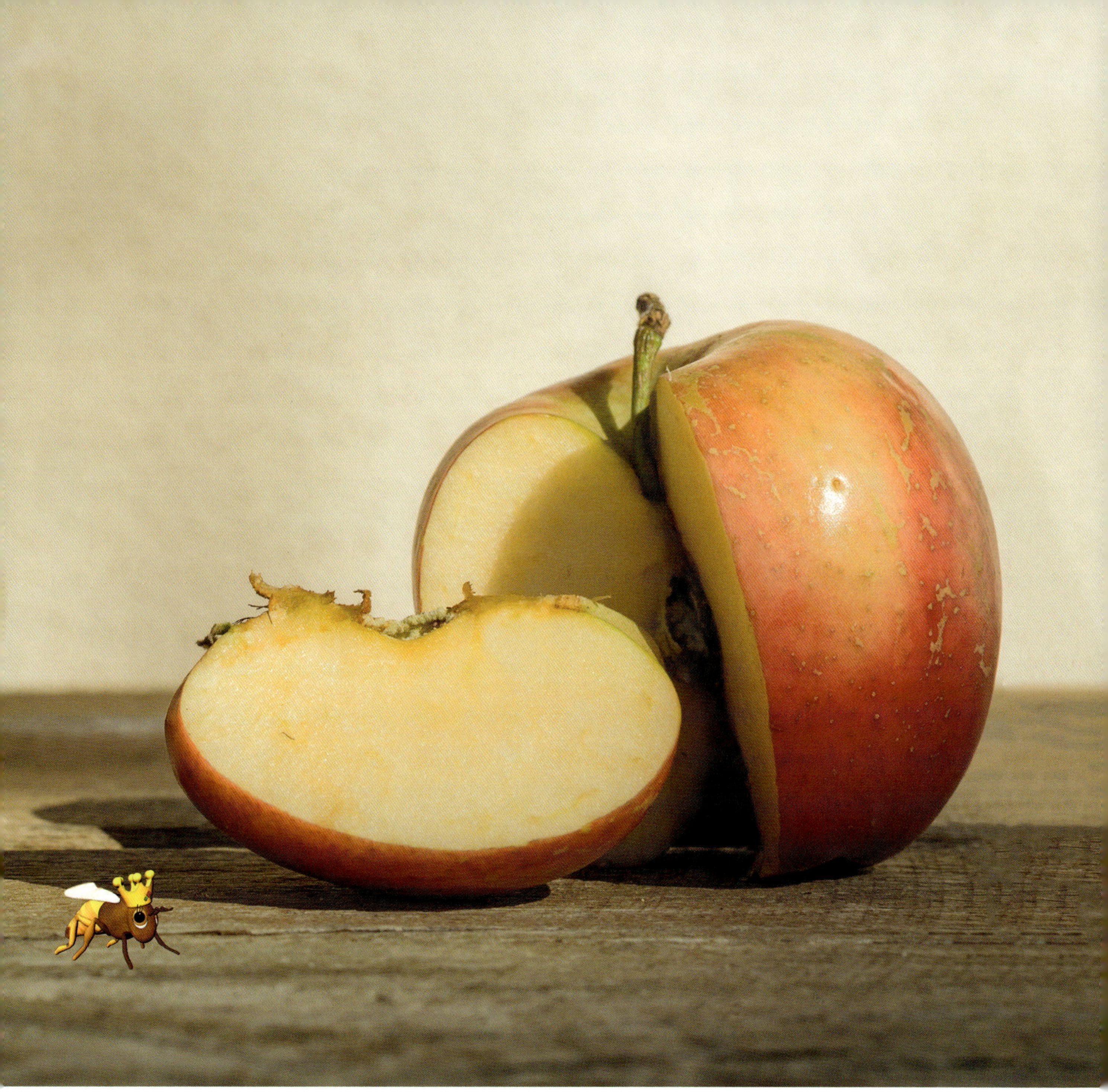

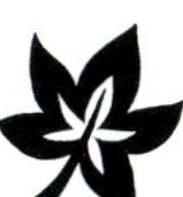

In Season
Autumn

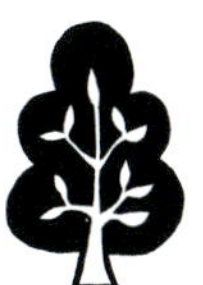

Grows How?
In trees

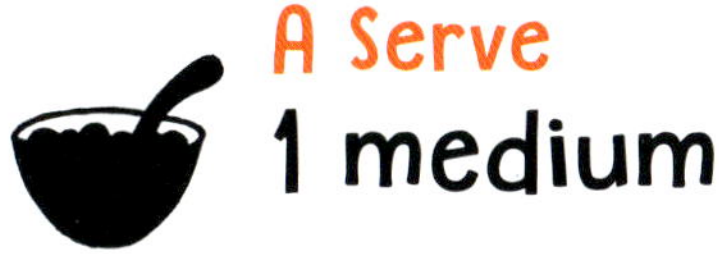

A Serve
1 medium

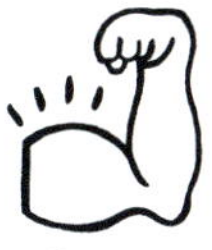

Good For Your
strength

tummy

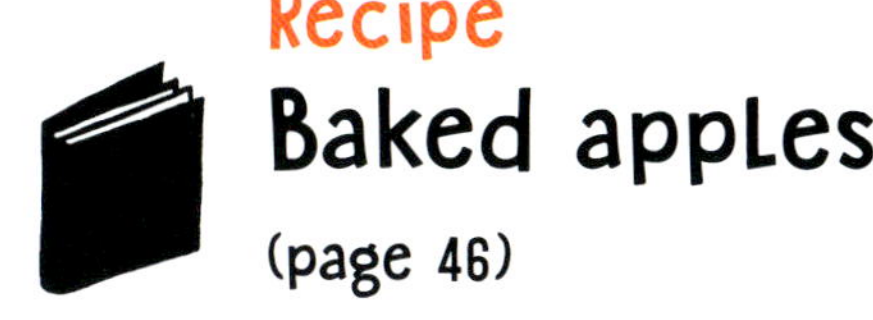

Recipe
Baked apples
(page 46)

KIWI FRUIT

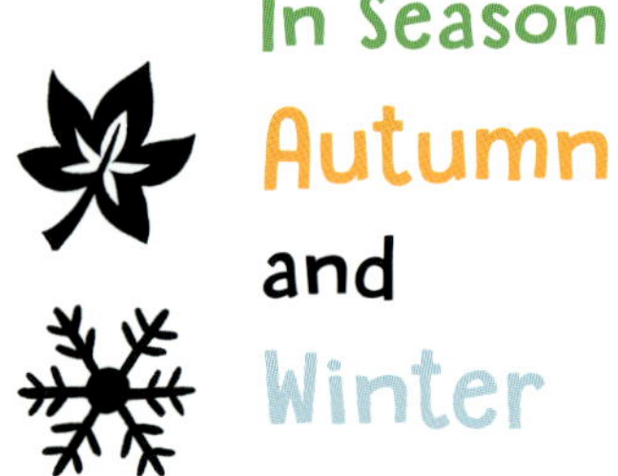

In Season

Autumn

and

Winter

Grows How?

On vines

A Serve

2 small or 1 large

Good For Your

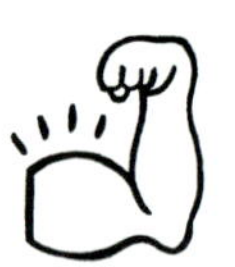

strength

heart

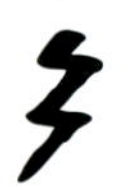

energy

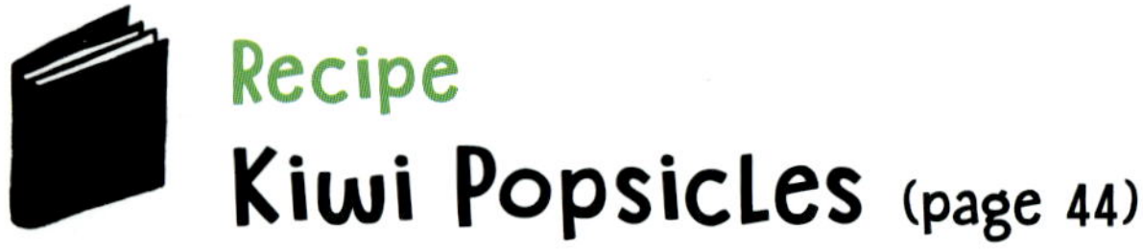

Recipe

Kiwi Popsicles (page 44)

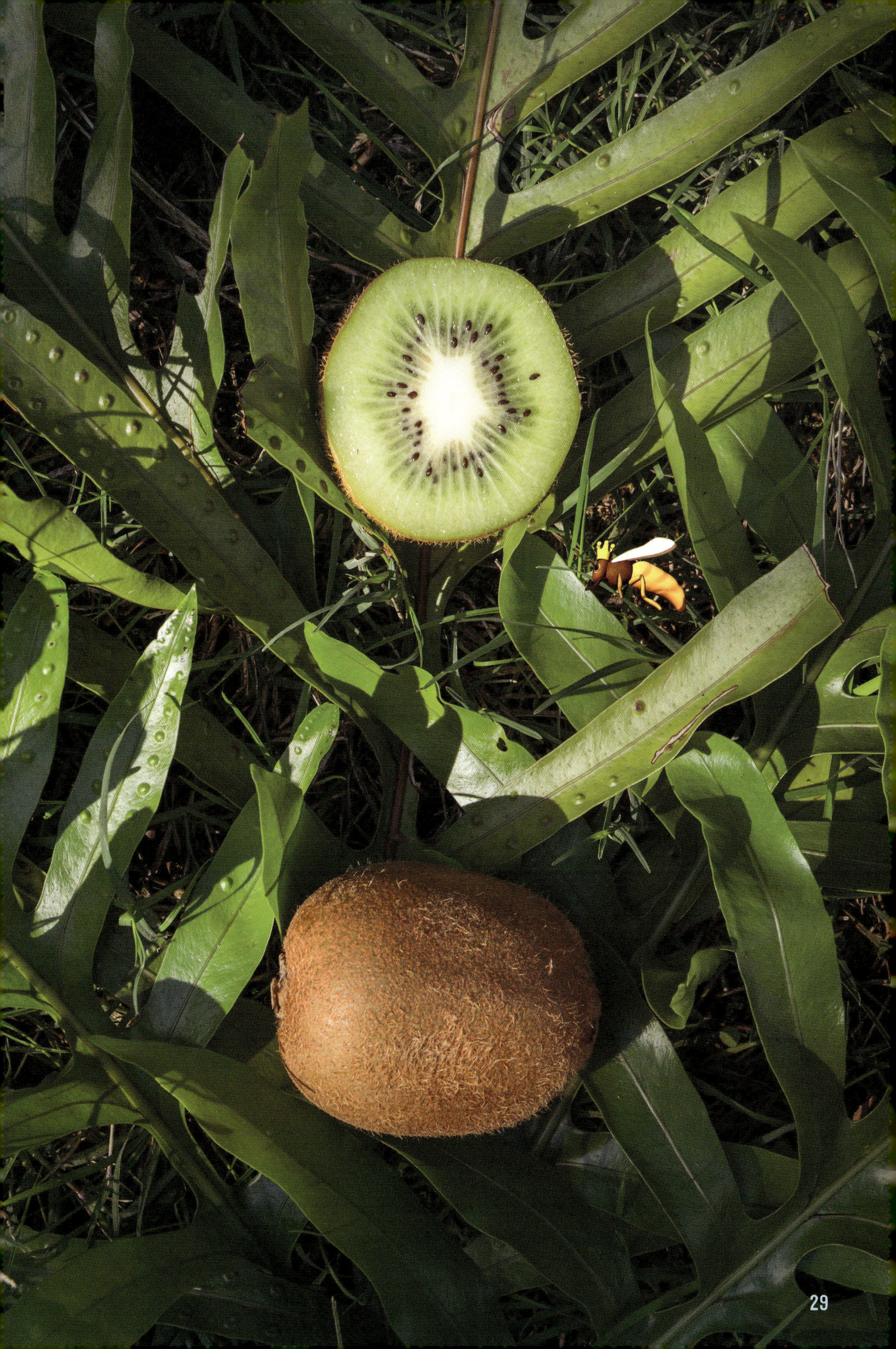

MANDARINS

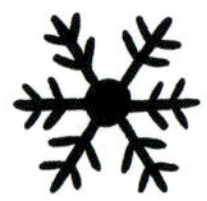

In Season

Winter

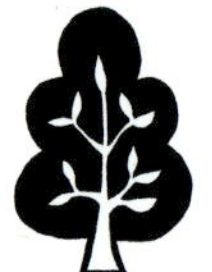

Grows How?

In trees

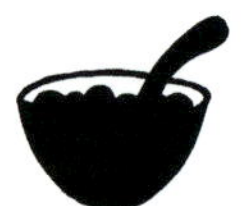

A Serve

2 small or 1 large

Good For Your

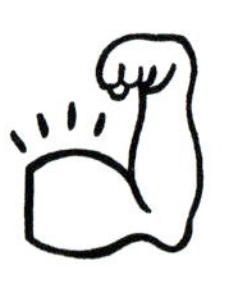

strength

heart

Recipe

Mandarin Salad (page 45)

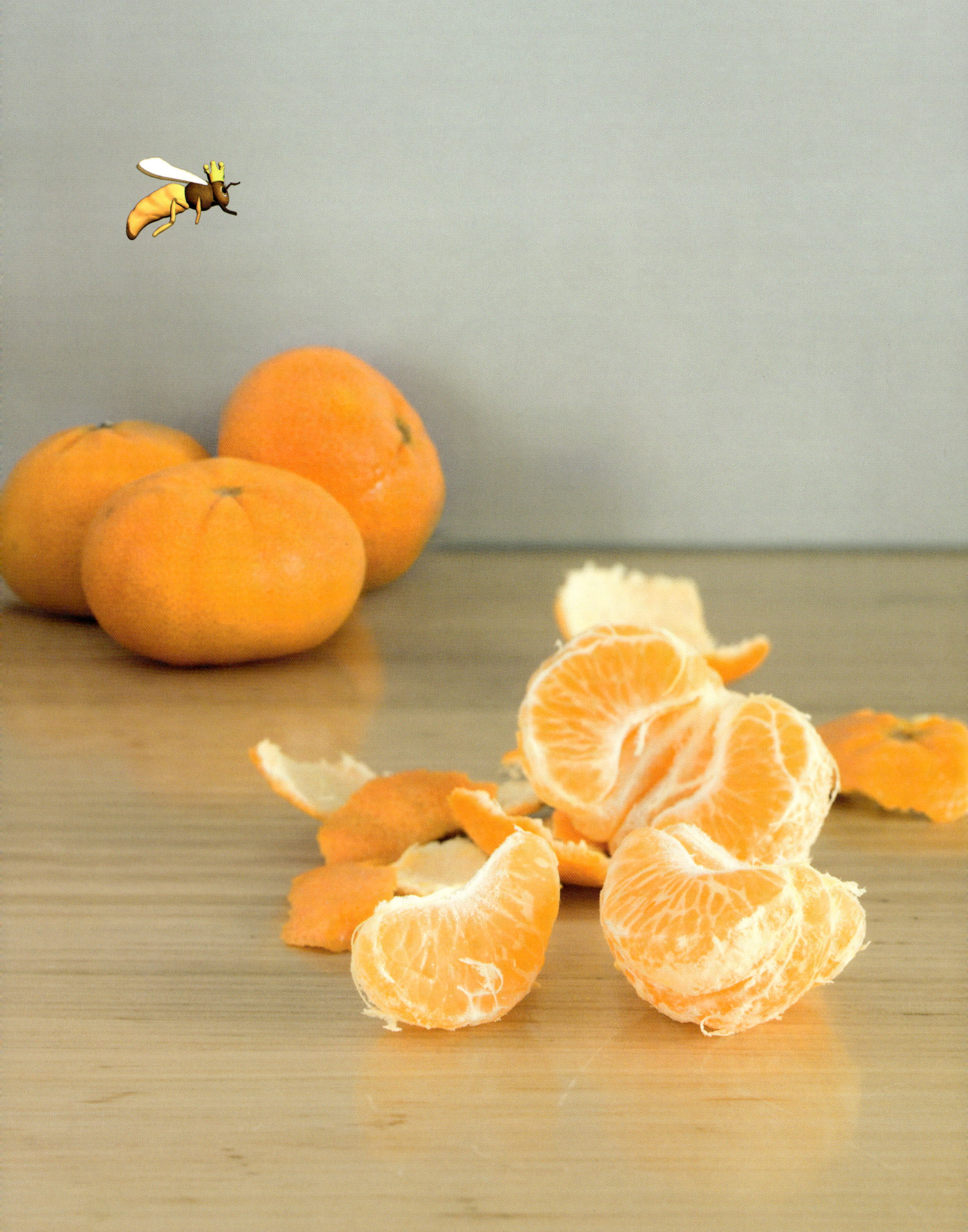

LEMON/LIME

In Season

 Spring, 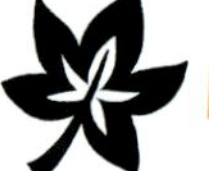 Autumn and 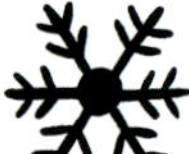 Winter (Lemons)

 Summer and 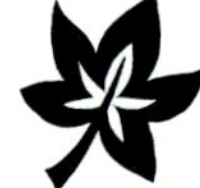 Autumn (Limes)

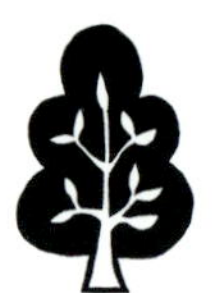

Grows How?

In trees

A Serve

1 medium

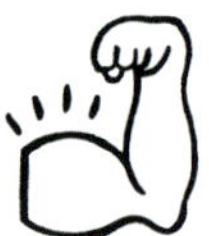

Good For Your

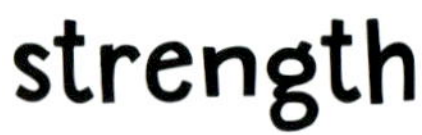

strength

 heart

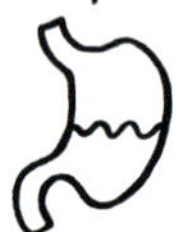 tummy

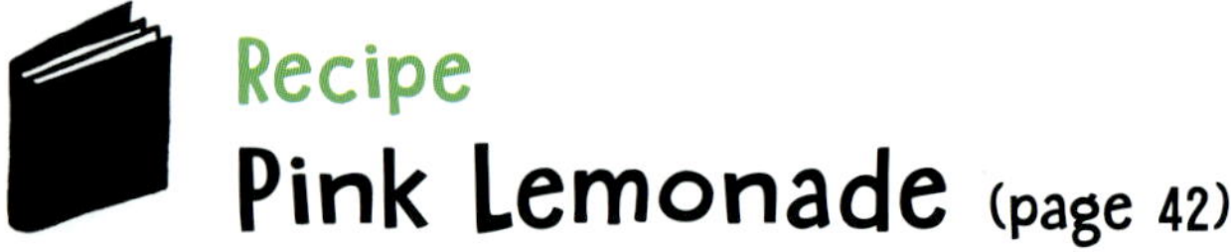

Recipe

Pink Lemonade (page 42)

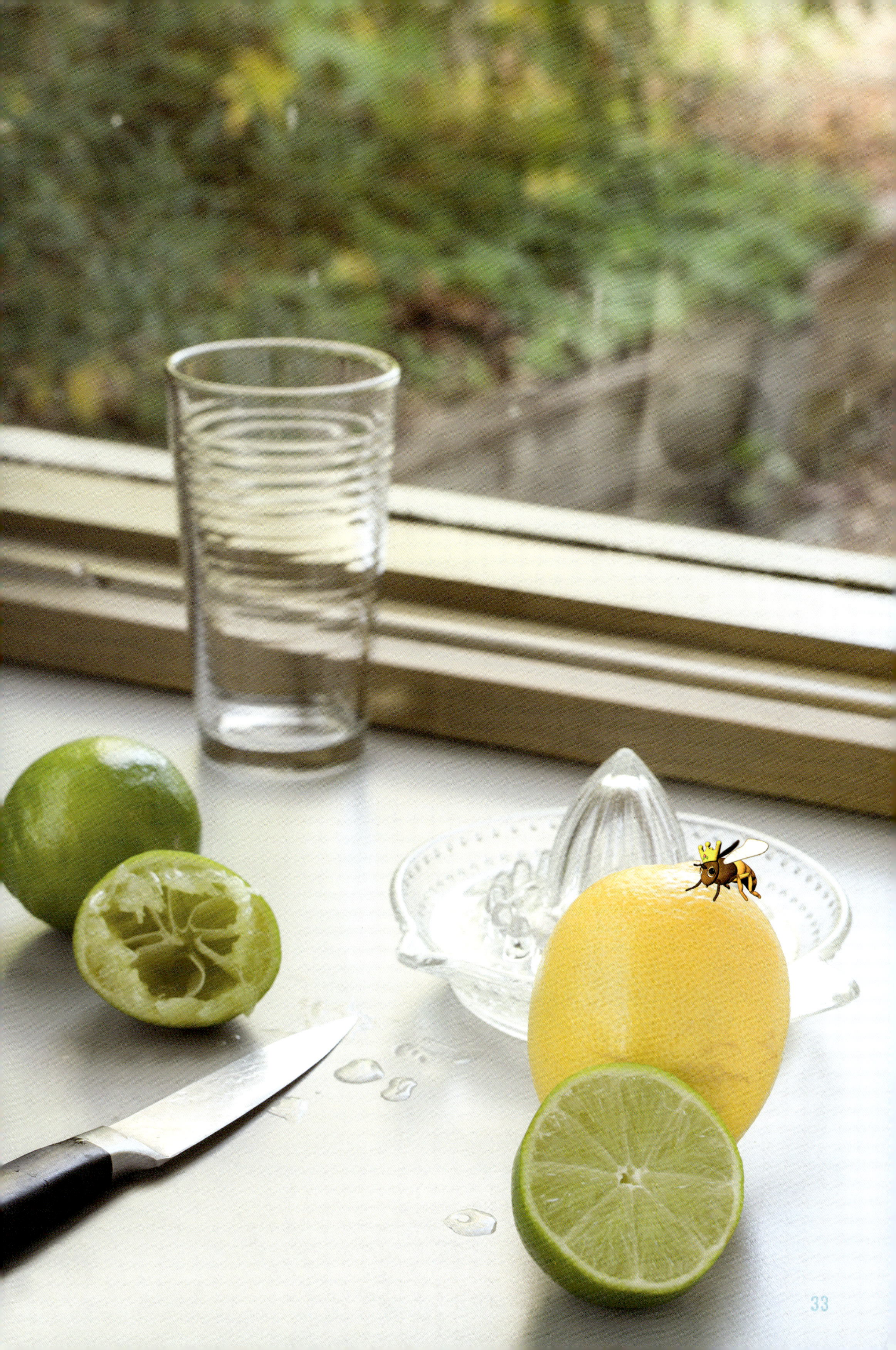

BANANA

In Season

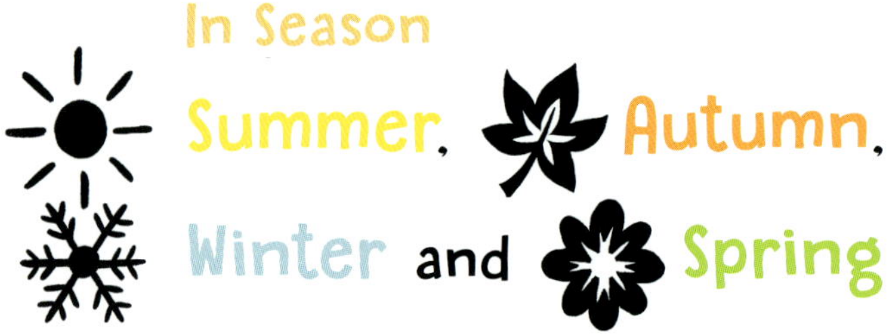

Summer, Autumn, Winter and Spring

Grows How?

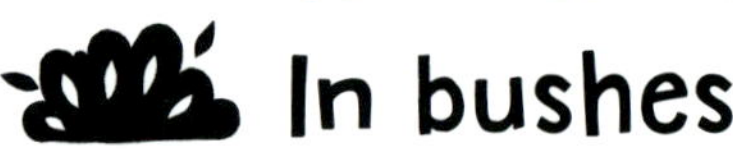

In bushes

A Serve

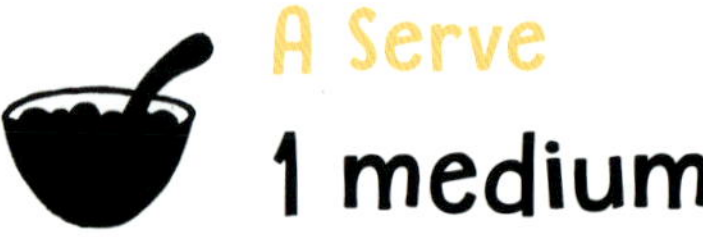

1 medium

Good For Your

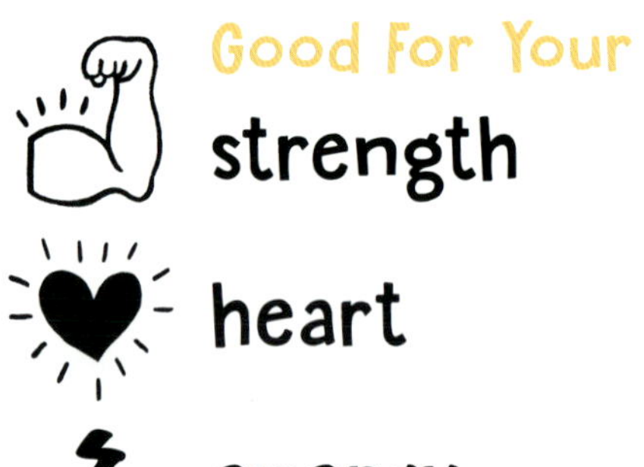

strength

heart

energy

Recipe

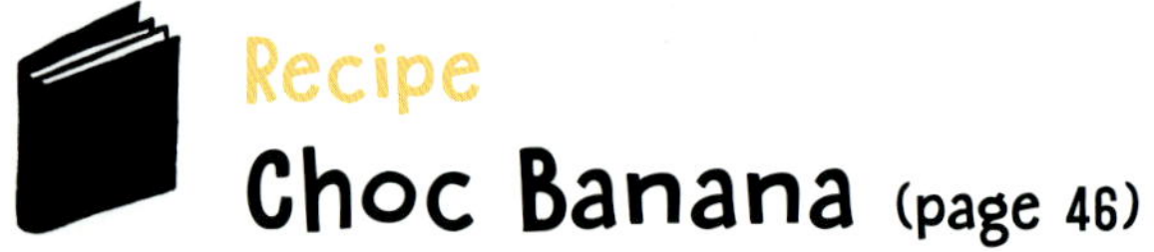

Choc Banana (page 46)

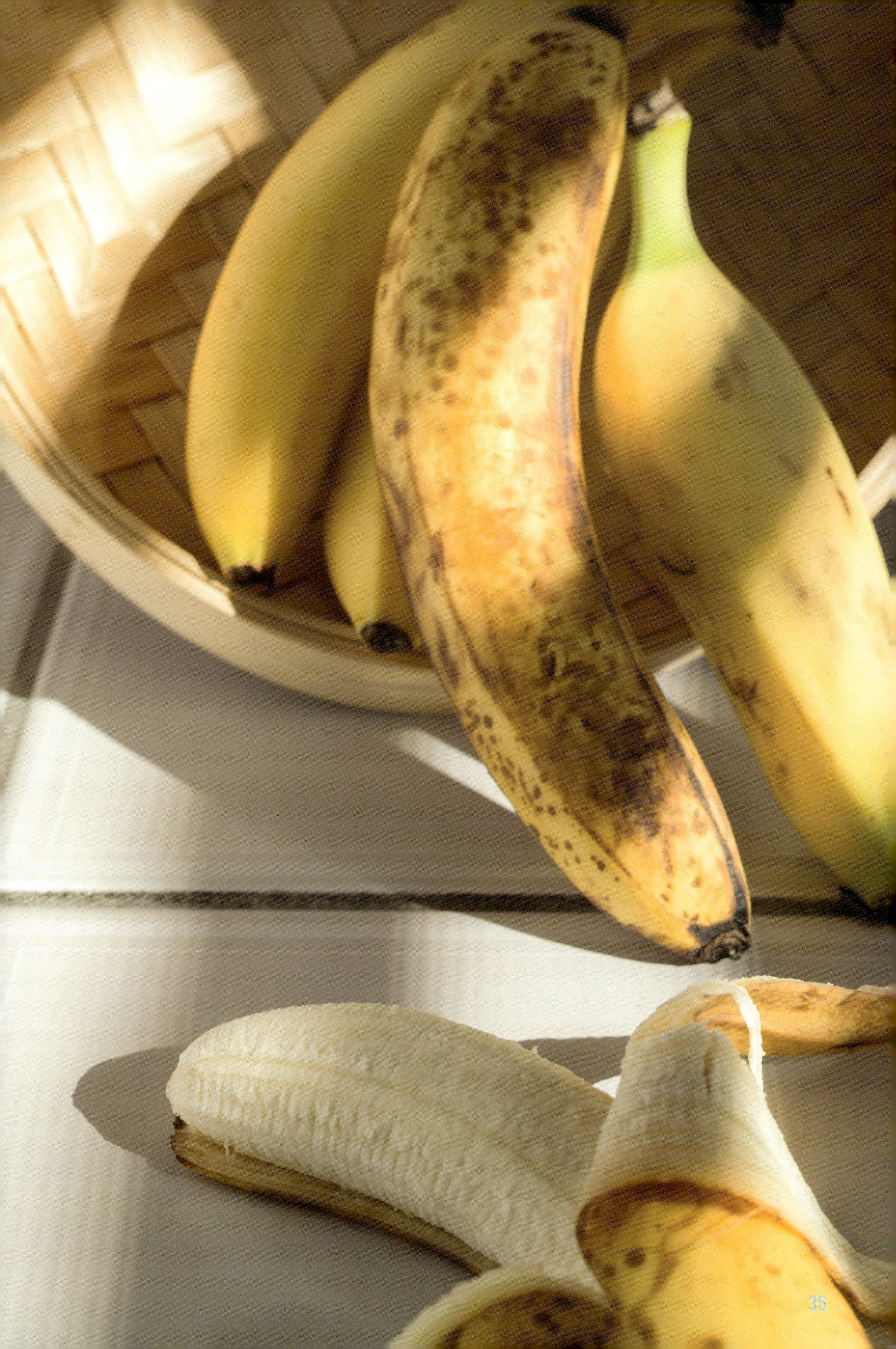

AVOCADO

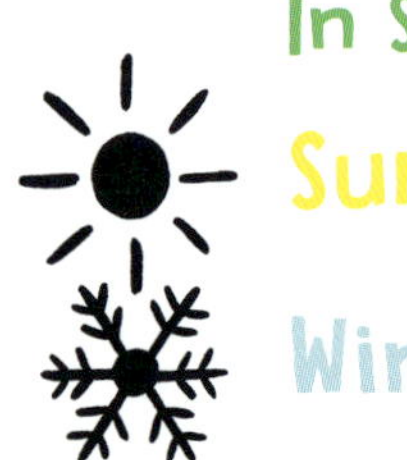

In Season

Summer, 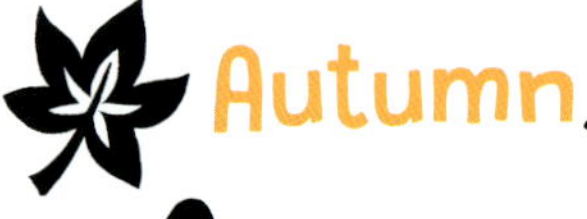 Autumn,

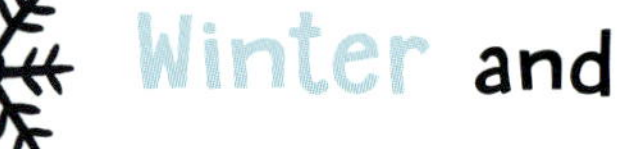 Winter and 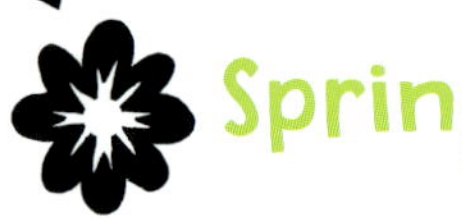 Spring

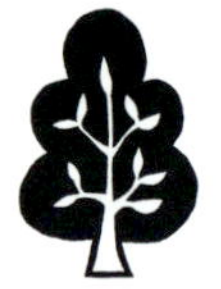

Grows How?

In trees

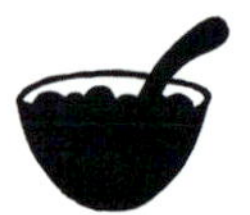

A Serve

1/3 medium avocado

Good For Your

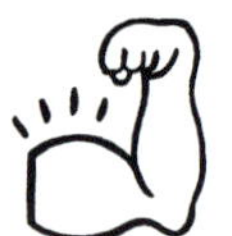

strength

heart

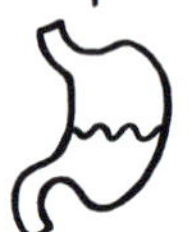

tummy

Recipe

Avocado and Basil Bruschetta (page 40)

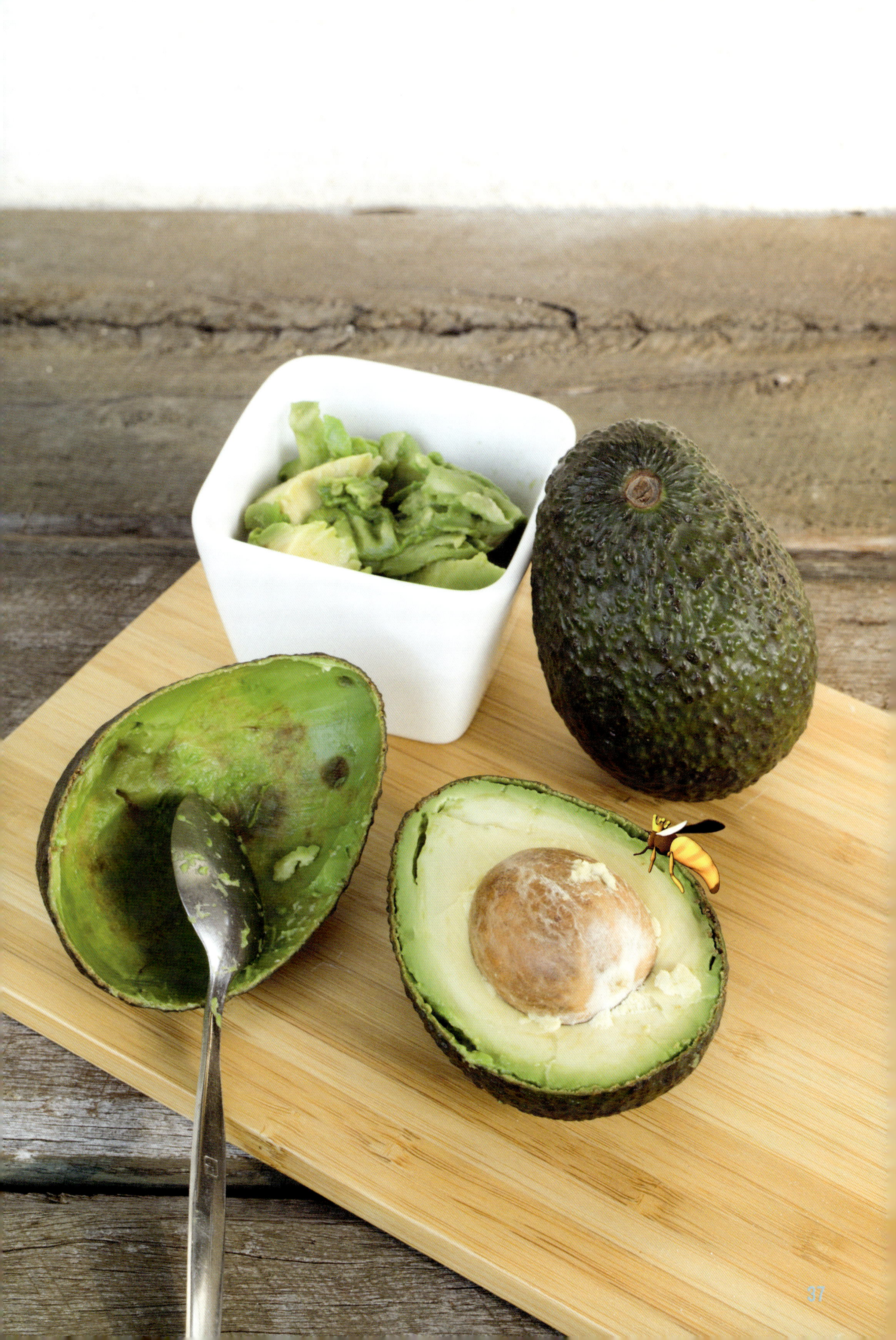

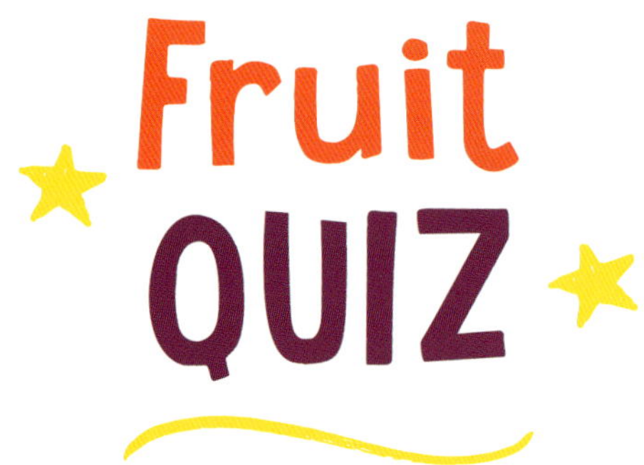

Let's see if you can answer some of the questions in the box below?

It's ok if you don't know the answers, just go back through the book and find them.

1 How much fruit should **YOU** eat each day?

2 Name all the **seasons** of the year.

3 Name 3 ways **fruit HELPS** you.

4 Where do **apples** grow?

5 Where do **kiwi fruit** grow?

6 What seasons do **bananas** grow?

ANSWERS

Answer 1: 4-8 yrs — 1½ serves of fruit; 9-11+ yrs — 2 serves of fruit.

Answer 2: Summer, Autumn, Winter, Spring.

Answer 3: Strength, eyes, tummy, bones, heart, brain.

Answer 4: on a tree

Answer 5: on a vine

Answer 6: All seasons!

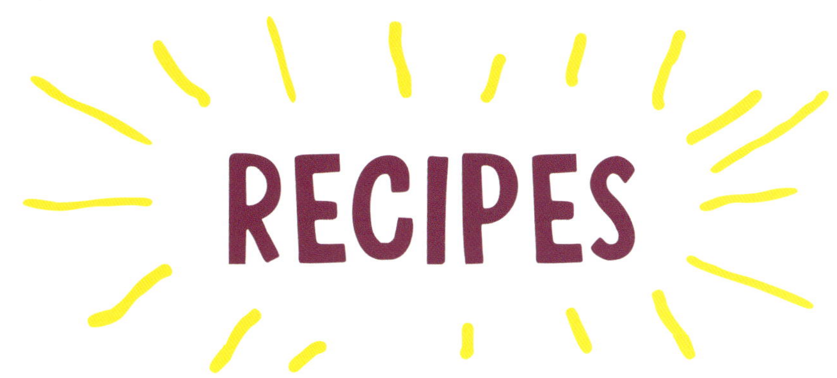

All of these recipes are classed as EASY. However, they are not for children. Adults can work with children to complete the recipes, but the adult is ultimately responsible for safety in the kitchen.

The coloured lines of the method are tasks you might look to ask your child to help with.

There is a note under each heading of how to choose the fruit when shopping and how to store it at home.

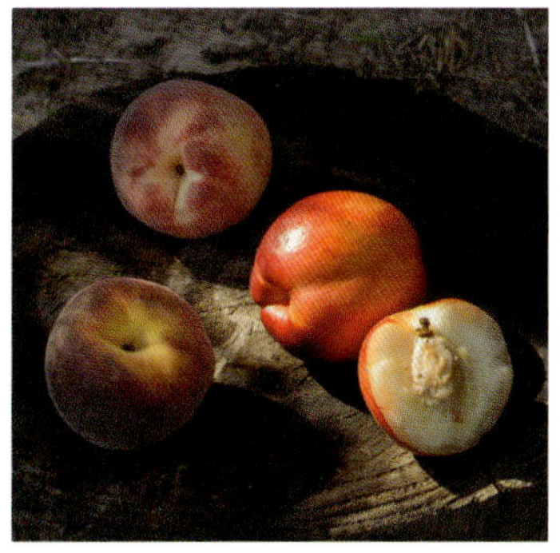

STONE FRUIT (page 20)

How to store:

At room temperature until ripe, then in the fridge.

How to choose:

The fruit must give slightly to the touch. Smell it and avoid bruises/cuts.

NECTARINE (APRICOT, PLUM, OR PEACH) AND YOGHURT SLICE

- 150g butter
- 2 eggs (room temp)
- ½ cup caster sugar
- 1 ½ cups wholemeal self raising flour
- ¼ tsp bi carb soda
- 1 tsp vanilla essence
- 1 tsp ground cinnamon
- 1 cup plain greek yoghurt
- ½ cup almonds, chopped
- 4 fresh nectarines, stones removed and sliced into quarters

a) Preheat oven 180 degrees Celsius. Line baking tray 20 x 30cm with baking paper.

b) Blend butter and sugar in blender until white. Add in eggs one at a time.

c) Sift flour with bi carb and cinnamon.

d) Fold yoghurt and flour through egg mixture. Add in vanilla essence. Fold through ¾ fruit and all nuts gently.

e) Spoon mix into tray and flatten until smooth. Top with remaining fruit pieces.

f) Bake for 20-25 minutes until skewer comes out clean. Leave in tray for 5 minutes before transferring to cooling rack. Remove paper to serve.

One cube of 3cm x 3cm is a serve.

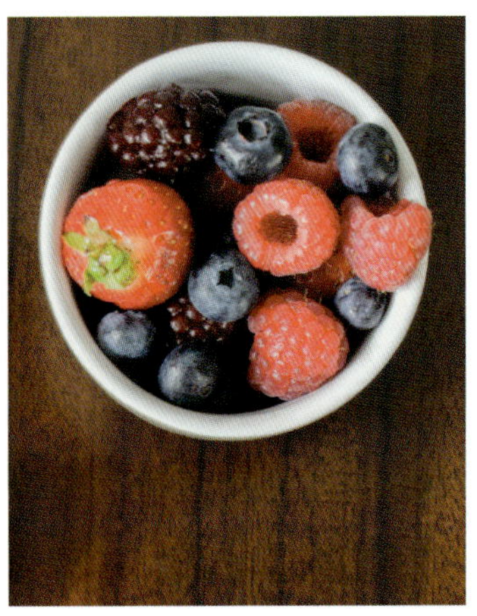

BERRIES (STRAWBERRIES, BLUEBERRIES, BLACKBERRIES, RASPBERRIES) (page 8)

How to store:

Not for long! Store in a shallow dish, single layer only, in the fridge. Wash just before eating, not before storing. You don't want them to be wet.

How to choose:

Berries of most types are best when they are a full color that is dark/deep.

BERRY COMPOTE

3 cups fresh or frozen berries

3 tablespoons freshly squeezed orange juice

¼ tsp cinnamon

¼ tsp clove or cardamom

a) Put all ingredients into a small pot.

b) Boil on low heat for 4-5 minutes.

c) Let sit and cool, then transfer into an air tight container for storage in the refrigerator for topping on porridge or pancakes or to mix with plain greek yoghurt for a healthy dessert.

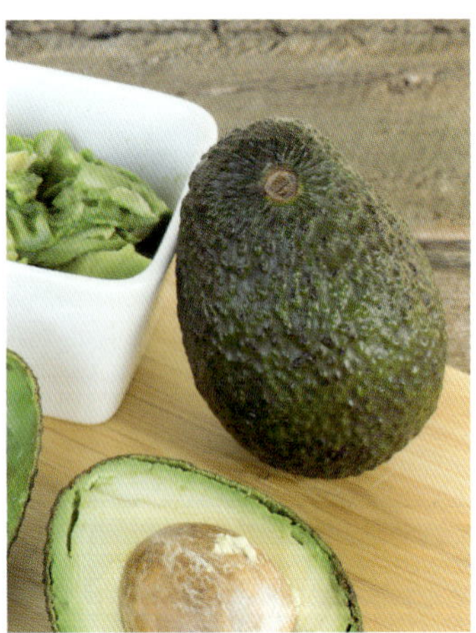

AVOCADO (page 36)

How to store:

Ripe: in the fridge; unripe, at room temperature. Once you cut it, best to squeeze lemon juice on it and store in air tight container to stop the browning.

How to choose:

If you want it ripe and ready to eat, you want it to "give" slightly with a light squeeze. If you want to eat it in 4-5 days, you can buy it firm and wait for it to darken up/ripen.

AVOCADO AND BASIL BRUSCHETTA

1 large firm avocado, diced

Handful of shredded washed basil leaves

1 punnet cherry tomatoes, washed and halved

1 tsp olive oil

Juice from one lemon

4 slices of toasted grain bread

a) Toss all ingredients excluding bread in a bowl.

b) Serve on top of toast.

Serves 2 adults or 4 kids.

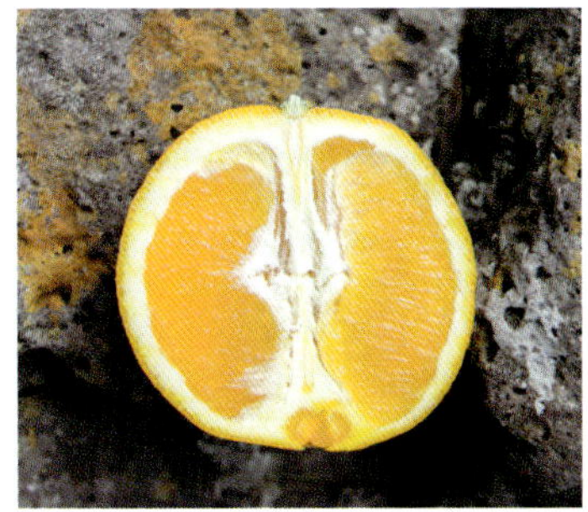

ORANGE (page 14)

How to store:

At room temperature.

How to choose:

Smell it! Tender texture; wrinkles on the skin is good, heavy for its size great!

ORANGE AND BEETROOT SALAD

- 2 chopped oranges, segments in halves
- 2 tablespoons olive oil
- Pepper to taste
- 1 tablespoon orange juice
- 800g canned baby beetroots, drained and chopped in quarters
- 400g canned or fresh chickpeas, drained
- ½ cup toasted walnut halves
- 2 spring onions sliced
- 2 large handfuls of washed rocket
- 100g crumbled feta

a) Mix all ingredients except feta.

b) Top salad with feta, season to taste. .

Serves 2 as main or 4 as a side.

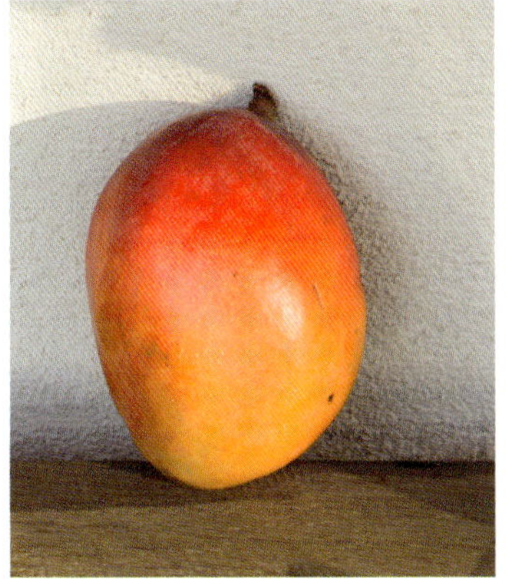

MANGO (page 12)

How to store:

Mangoes that are hard can be stored in a paper bag for a few days or just left out of the sun at room temperature. Once fully ripe, they can be stored in the fridge for a few days.

How to choose:

Smell it! it should be fragrant and firm and give slightly to the touch.

MANGO LASSI

- 500g mango roughly chopped
- 250g greek plain yoghurt
- 2 tsp melted or runny honey

a) Put all ingredients into a blender.

b) Blend until smooth.

Serves 4.

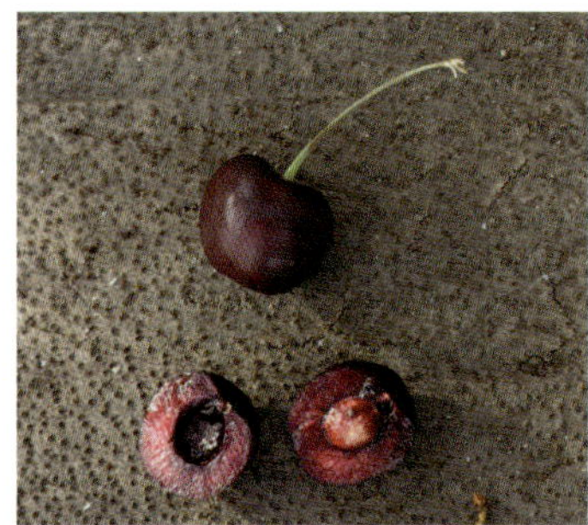

CHERRY (page 18)

How to store:

in an air tight container in the fridge.

How to choose:

Firm, shiny skins, heavy and deep in color. A green stem is better than a dry/woody stem.

CHERRY SALAD

Dressing:

4 tablespoons of extra virgin olive oil

Juice from one fresh lemon

½ tsp cracked pepper

Salad:

4 cups of fresh baby spinach, roughly chopped

1 cup of fresh cherries pitted, chopped

½ a red onion thinly sliced

¼ cup of shelled pistachios, chopped

¼ cup of crumbled feta

Dressing:

a) Add ingredients to medium bowl and whisk to combine.

Salad:

b) Add all ingredients to a bowl.

c) Top with dressing, toss and serve.

Serves 4 as a side.

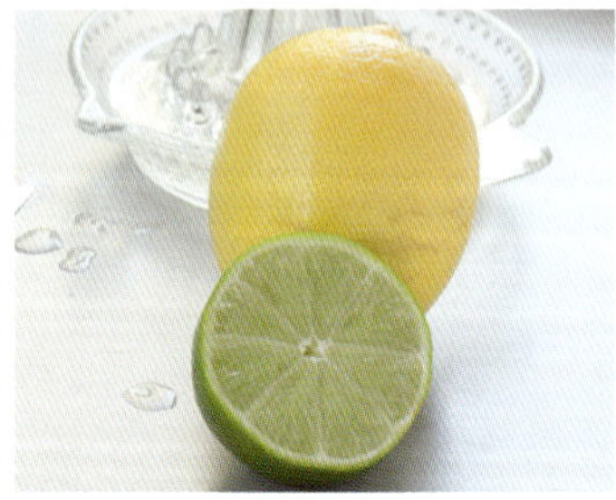

LEMON / LIME (page 32)

How to store:

At room temperature. They start to shrink when overripe.

How to choose:

A deep colour, heavy, firm wrinkle free skin and nice smell.

PINK LEMONADE

1 ½ cups lemon juice

3/4 cup caster sugar

4 cups boiling water

Berry mix

70g fresh or frozen raspberries

2 tsp caster sugar

Handful of mint

Slices of lemon

a) Boil lemon juice, water and sugar until sugar is dissolved.

b) Refrigerate.

c) Boil berries and 2 tsp caster sugar until dissolved. Refrigerate.

d) Add berries to lemon juice mix then sieve into a serving jug.

e) Add mint and lemon to serve with ice cubes.

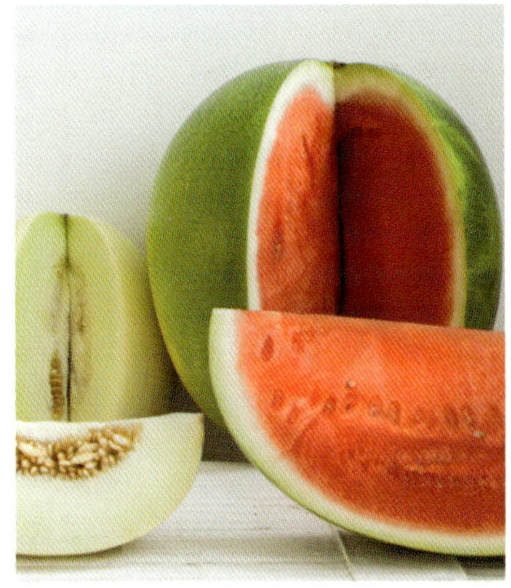

MELON (HONEYDEW, CANTALOUPE AND WATERMELON) (page 10)

How to store:

At room temperature if uncut. In fridge as soon as cut.

How to choose:

Avoid any melons with cuts or bruising. Smell the melon; push the blossom end (opposite to the stem) and if it yields slightly to pressure, it is ripe. You want a heavy melon!

WATERMELON SALAD

- 3 cups chopped watermelon, large chunks
- 300g cherry tomatoes, halved
- 200g goats cheese, crumbed
- Handful of basil, roughly chopped
- ½ cup toasted pistachios
- 1 tablespoon balsamic vinegar mixed with 2 tablespoons extra virgin olive oil

a) Place melon and pistachio on plate.
b) Mix tomatoes with basil, oil and balsamic.
c) Top melon with tomato/basil mix.
d) Top all of salad with crumbed cheese.

Serves 4 as a side.

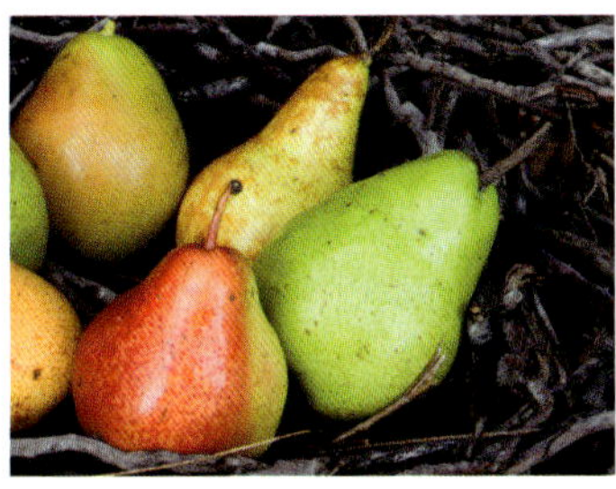

PEARS (page 24)

How to store:

At room temperature until ripe and then in the fridge

How to choose:

A ripe pear gives a little under pressure at the stem end.

PEAR, PUMPKIN AND WALNUT SALAD

- 2 brown pears, sliced
- 4 large handfuls of washed & dried rocket
- ½ cup toasted walnuts
- ½ butternut pumpkin, sliced, leave skin on
- 1 red onion sliced
- 100g feta crumbed
- 1 tablespoon balsamic vinegar
- 2 tablespoons extra virgin olive oil

a) Grill onion and pumpkin with 1 tablespoon oil until cooked. Cool.
b) Toss rocket, nuts and cooled pumpkin/onion. Place pears and cheese on top. Drizzle oil and vinegar. Lightly toss and season to taste.

Serves 4 as a side.

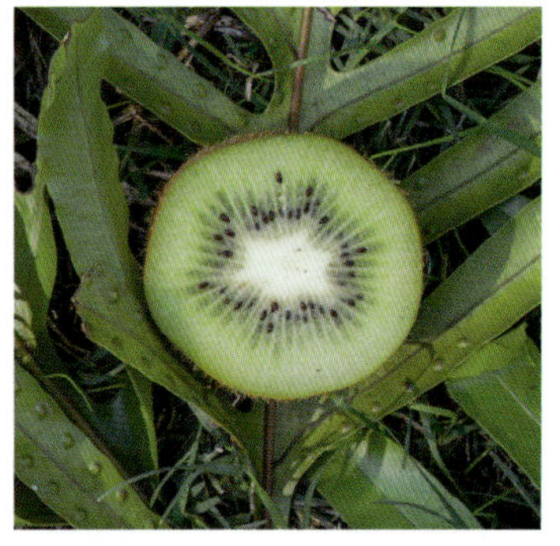

KIWI FRUIT (page 28)

How to store:

They ripen at room temperature; then store in the fridge for weeks, away from other fruits like apples.

How to choose:

Plump, smooth skin free of wrinkles, slightly give to pressure at the ends.

KIWI POPSICLES

8-10 kiwi fruit, puree, skin off

1.5 cups mango or pineapple juice, no added sugar

2 tsp honey

a) Put all ingredients into a blender: and blend all ingredients, then put into popsicles and freeze.

b) As above, but instead of mango juice/honey add in 1 can light coconut cream and 1 tablespoon brown sugar.

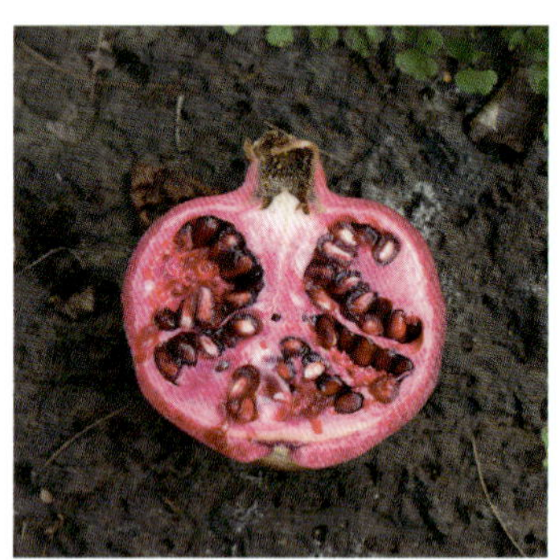

POMEGRANATE (page 22)

How to store:

A ripe one at room temperature for a few days but then in a bag/air tight container in the fridge for up to 3 months.

How to choose:

You want it to be heavy and dark, with no cracks, bruises or puckering when you rub it. Skin should be tight.

BULGER AND POMEGRANATE SALAD

1 cup bulger

1 cup boiling water

1 cup pomegranate seeds

½ cup mint leaves

½ cup parsley leaves

2 tablespoons lemon juice

¼ cup sultanas or raisins

3 tablespoons extra virgin olive oil

300g cherry tomato halved

¼ cup chopped almonds, toasted

3 spring onions thinly sliced

a) Cover bulger with boiling water. Cover with lid until bulger absorbs water (around 30 minutes).

b) Mix all other ingredients into a bowl, add bulger.

Serves 4 as a side.

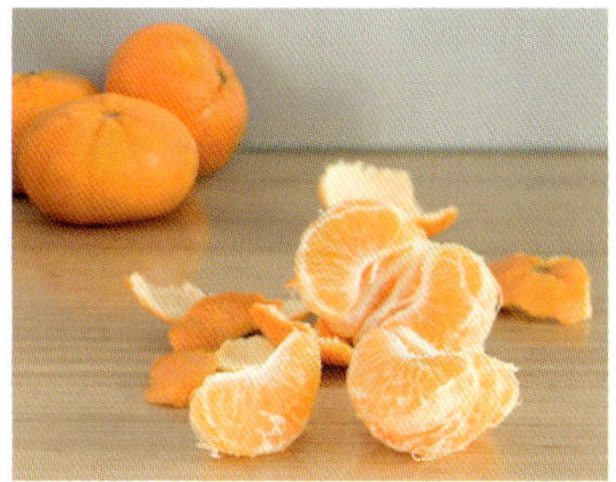

MANDARINS (page 30)

How to store:

In cool dark areas or in the fridge.

How to choose:

Heavy and glossy.

MANDARIN SALAD

4 seedless mandarins, segmented and sliced longways in half

1 large red capsicum, deseeded, thinly sliced

2 large carrots, coarsely grated

60g snow pea sprouts, trimmed

3 shallots, trimmed, sliced

⅔ cup (90g) pecans, thinly sliced

1 tablespoon sesame seeds, toasted

Dressing:

1 ½ tablespoons extra virgin olive oil

1 tablespoon red wine vinegar

2 teaspoons honey

3cm piece fresh ginger, finely grated

a) Combine all dressing ingredients and mix. Pour over salad.

Serves 4 as a side.

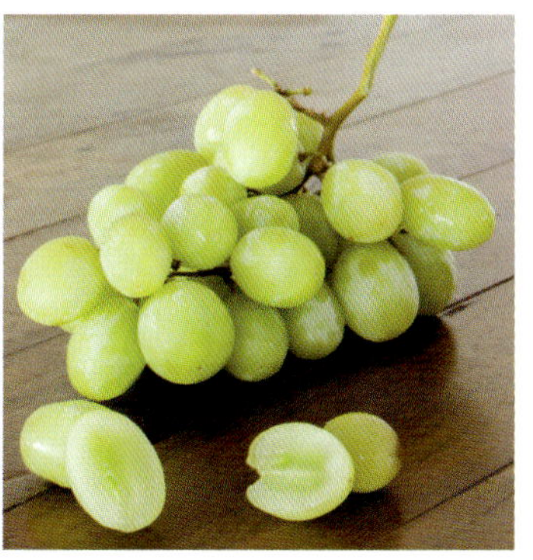

GRAPES (page 16)

How to store:

In the refrigerator, in a bag or air tight container, unwashed. Wash before eating!

How to choose:

Colour: red grapes should be deep red and green, dark green. Ensure they are nice and plump and not falling off their stems.

FROZEN GRAPES!

On skewers or in a packet

a) Wash and dry before freezing. Freeze whole grapes, in single layers on baking paper, or on a skewer, then use to cool drinks or blend for a frozen drink.

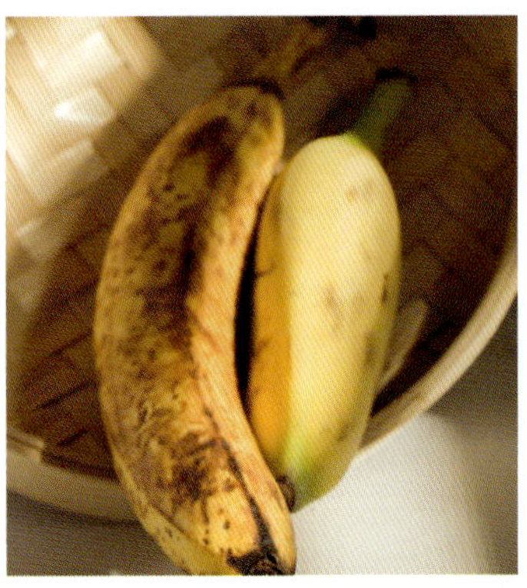

BANANA (page 34)

How to store:

At room temperature with other fruits until all yellow or even with some brown spots. Once ripe, you must eat it, or peel and put in freezer container for cooking with later.

How to choose:

A ripe banana has no green, it is all yellow. Once it is more brown than yellow, it is over ripe.

CHOC BANANAS

- 4 ripe bananas
- 200g dark chocolate
- Shredded coconut, chopped nuts and sprinkles
- 4 skewers for bananas (can be ice pole sticks, kebab skewers or even straws)

a) Skewer ripe skinned bananas. Place on baking paper and place flat in the freezer to freeze overnight or at least 3 hours.

b) Melt dark chocolate in glass bowl in microwave on high for 1 minute. Stir, then repeat in 30 second intervals until melted.

c) Dip bananas into chocolate and then roll in coconut/nuts/sprinkles. Put back in freezer until chocolate has gone hard. Enjoy!

One banana is a serve.

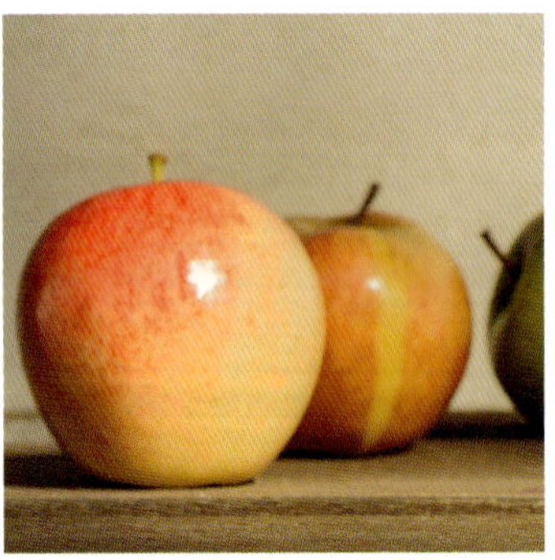

APPLES (page 26)

How to store:

At room temperature.

How to choose:

Apples are ready for eating as soon as they are off the tree! You can tell if they are not good for eating, with bruising, cuts or worms!

BAKED APPLES

- Apples x 4 (green), whole and cored
- Juice from one lemon
- ⅓ cup sultanas
- tablespoons x2 slivered almonds toasted
- 2 tsp mixed spice
- 2 tsp vanilla essence
- 1 tablespoon brown sugar

a) Pre heat oven to 180 degrees.

b) Core apples, place in baking tray and put lemon juice into cored hole.

c) Mix all other ingredients and teaspoon into apple holes.

d) Cover with foil and bake for 10-15 minutes

e) Remove foil and bake for 10 minutes more.

f) Serve warm with custard.

Serves 4.